Rural and Other Medically Underserved Populations

Editors

JOANN S. OLIVER
SANDRA MILLON UNDERWOOD

NURSING CLINICS
OF NORTH AMERICA

www.nursing.theclinics.com

Consulting Editor
STEPHEN D. KRAU

September 2015 • Volume 50 • Number 3

ELSEVIER

1600 John F. Kennedy Boulevard • Suite 1800 • Philadelphia, Pennsylvania, 19103-2899

http://www.theclinics.com

NURSING CLINICS OF NORTH AMERICA Volume 50, Number 3
September 2015 ISSN 0029-6465, ISBN-13: 978-0-323-39573-1

Editor: Kerry Holland
Developmental Editor: Casey Jackson

Nursing Clinics of North America (ISSN 0029-6465) is published quarterly by Elsevier Inc., 360 Park Avenue South, New York, NY 10010-1710. Months of Issue are March, June, September, and December. Periodicals postage paid at New York, NY and additional mailing offices. Subscription price per year is, $150.00 (US individuals), $400.00 (US institutions), $275.00 (international individuals), $488.00 (international institutions), $220.00 (Canadian individuals), $488.00 (Canadian institutions), $85.00 (US students), and $135.00 (international students). To receive student/resident rate, orders must be accompanied by name of affiliated institution, date of term, and the signature of program/residency coordinator on institution letterhead. Orders will be billed at individual rate until proof of status is received. Foreign air speed delivery is included in all *Clinics* subscription prices. All prices are subject to change without notice. **POSTMASTER:** Send address changes to *Nursing Clinics*, Elsevier Health Sciences Division, Subscription Customer Service, 3251 Riverport Lane, Maryland Heights, MO 63043. **Customer Service: Telephone: 1-800-654-2452** (U.S. and Canada); **1-314-447-8871 (outside U.S. and Canada). Fax: 1-314-447-8029. E-mail: journalscustomerservice-usa@elsevier.com** (for print support) and **journalsonlinesupport-usa@elsevier.com** (for online support).

Nursing Clinics of North America is covered in *EMBASE/Excerpta Medica, MEDLINE/PubMed (Index Medicus), Social Sciences Citation Index, Current Contents, ASCA, Cumulative Index to Nursing, RNdex Top 100,* and Allied Health Literature and International Nursing Index (INI).

Contributors

CONSULTING EDITOR

STEPHEN D. KRAU, PhD, RN, CNE
Associate Professor, Vanderbilt University Medical Center, School of Nursing, Nashville, Tennessee

EDITORS

JOANN S. OLIVER, PhD, RN, CNE
Associate Professor, The University of Alabama, Capstone College of Nursing, Tuscaloosa, Alabama

SANDRA MILLON UNDERWOOD, PhD, RN, FAAN
Professor, University of Wisconsin Milwaukee, College of Nursing, Milwaukee, Wisconsin

AUTHORS

ELIZABETH ALLEY
The University of Alabama, Tuscaloosa, Alabama

DANIEL M. AVERY Jr, MD
College of Community Health Sciences, University of Alabama, Tuscaloosa, Alabama

SPENCER BAER
The University of Alabama, Tuscaloosa, Alabama

JANELLE R. BAKER, PhD, APRN, A-GPCNP-BC
Associate Professor, Associate Dean and Director, Graduate Nursing Programs, Alcorn State University, Natchez, Mississippi

LAWANDA W. BASKIN, MSN, APRN, FNP-C
Assistant Professor, Graduate Nursing Programs, Alcorn State University, Natchez, Mississippi

MARGARET T. BOWERS, DNP, RN, FNP-BC, FAANP
Duke University School of Nursing and Duke Division of Cardiology, Durham, North Carolina

TERESA L. BRYAN, MSN, APRN, FNP-BC
Assistant Professor, Program Coordinator, FNP Track, Alcorn State University, Natchez, Mississippi

DONNA CALVIN, PhD, FNP-BC
Assistant Professor, Department of Nursing, Governors State University, University Park, Illinois

MARY K. CANALES, PhD, RN
Professor, Department of Nursing, University of Wisconsin-Eau Claire, Eau Claire, Wisconsin

HEATHER D. CARTER-TEMPLETON, PhD, RN-BC
Assistant Professor, Capstone College of Nursing, The University of Alabama, Tuscaloosa, Alabama

NANCY COFFEY, BA
Supplemental Nutrition Assistance Program Education (SNAP-Ed) Coordinator, University of Wisconsin Cooperative Extension, Eau Claire County, Altoona, Wisconsin

PATRICK EWELL, MA
Graduate Assistant, Department of Psychology, The University of Alabama, Tuscaloosa, Alabama

AUDWIN B. FLETCHER, PhD, APRN, FNP-BC, FAAN
University of Mississippi Medical School of Nursing, Jackson, Mississippi

MARILYN COOPER HANDLEY, RN, MSN, PhD
Capstone College of Nursing, The University of Alabama, Tuscaloosa, Alabama

EMILY A. HAOZOUS, PhD, RN
Assistant Professor, University of New Mexico College of Nursing, Albuquerque, New Mexico

PAIGE JOHNSON, PhD, RN
Assistant Professor, Capstone College of Nursing, The University of Alabama, Tuscaloosa, Alabama

REBECCA JOHNSON, MLIS
Instructional Design Researcher and Consultant, Rochester Institute of Technology, Rochester, New York

SHERYL KELBER, MA
Biostatistician and Information Specialist, Harriet H. Werley Center for Nursing Research and Evaluation, University of Wisconsin Milwaukee College of Nursing, Milwaukee, Wisconsin

MICHELLE LONG, MPH
Master of Public Health Program, University of Missouri, Columbia, Missouri

CHARLES E. MENIFIELD, MPA, PhD
Truman School of Public Affairs, University of Missouri, Columbia, Missouri

MICHELE MONTGOMERY, PhD, MPH, RN
Assistant Professor, Capstone College of Nursing, The University of Alabama, Tuscaloosa, Alabama

EMILY MOORE, BA
Executive Director, Feed My People Food Bank, Eau Claire, Wisconsin

CHARLES NEHER, BS
University of New Mexico, Albuquerque, New Mexico

JOANN S. OLIVER, PhD, RN, CNE
Associate Professor, The University of Alabama, Capstone College of Nursing, Tuscaloosa, Alabama

BARBARA D. POWE, PhD, RN, FAAN
Research Consultant, Lilburn, Georgia

YOLANDA M. POWELL-YOUNG, PhD, PCNS-BC, CPN
Professor, Dean, School of Nursing, Alcorn State University, Natchez, Mississippi

CANDY S. RINEHART, DNP, FNP, ADM-BC
Nurse Practitioner/Director of OSU Total Health and Wellness, Executive Director of Advance Practice and Community Partnerships, The Ohio State University College of Nursing, Columbus, Ohio

COSTELLIA H. TALLEY, PhD
Assistant Professor, College of Nursing, Michigan State University, East Lansing, Michigan

SANDRA MILLON UNDERWOOD, PhD, RN, FAAN
Professor, University of Wisconsin Milwaukee, College of Nursing, Milwaukee, Wisconsin

SANREKA R. WATLEY, MS
Account Executive, Unitron, Northern California, Hawaii

KAREN PATRICIA WILLIAMS, PhD
Associate Professor, Department of Obstetrics, Gynecology and Reproductive Biology, Michigan State University, East Lansing, Michigan

FELECIA G. WOOD, PhD, RN, CNL
Professor, The University of Alabama Capstone College of Nursing, Tuscaloosa, Alabama

LIN WU, MLIS, AHIP
Associate Professor, Health Sciences Librarian, Medical Science Library, A&M University, Kingsville, Texas

GERALDINE Q. YOUNG, DNP, FNP-BC
Assistant Professor, Graduate Nursing Programs, Alcorn State University, Natchez, Mississippi

Contents

Type 2 diabetes (T2DM) disproportionately affects the underserved population, and has been identified as the major risk factor for many microvascular diseases. T2DM also affects the vasculature and neural system of the inner ear, often leading to hearing loss, a major risk factor for falls, depression, and other health problems. This article aims to: increase awareness of the association between T2DM and hearing loss, promote screening for hearing loss, discuss available resources and assistive devices for those with hearing loss, and encourage nurses to take an active role in advocating for assessment and treatment of hearing loss in T2DM patients.

Despite general efforts to reduce risk factors in cardiovascular disease in the United States over the previous decade, disparities in cardiovascular care remain more prevalent in the underserved population. Recent focus has shifted from treatment of disease to promotion of health. The impact goals for 2020 are improvement in 7 health metrics (smoking status, body mass index, physical activity, healthy dietary score, total cholesterol, blood pressure, and fasting plasma glucose) of cardiovascular health and reduction of cardiovascular disease and stroke by 20%. Identification of those at high risk for poor cardiovascular health in adulthood should begin during early adolescence.

A focus group process, conducted by a community-academic partnership, qualitatively assessed food insecurity perspectives of parents and community staff assisting families with food assistance. Food insecurity was reported to affect all aspects of their life, increasing stress and reducing coping abilities. The Agency for Healthcare Research and Quality encourages research with priority populations, including low-income populations. This research supports the body of knowledge correlating relationships between poverty, food insecurity, and chronic health conditions. Perspectives of food-insecure people are often missing from policy and advocacy interventions. Nurses can use lessons learned and recommendations from this research to address food insecurity-related health disparities.

Health care spending is often addressed in discussions of budgeting and deficits in the United States. It is important to many Americans that funds allocated for health care spending be allocated and spent in the most efficient and effective manner, leading to improved health outcomes, particularly for underserved populations. Many studies address health care spending, but few address the issue of spending as it relates to societal well-being, or certain health outcomes that adversely impact communities. This study seeks to expand the available literature by analyzing data from national sources at the state level.

This article presents a review of the literature to identify best practices for clinical partnerships with indigenous populations of North America, specifically American Indian/Alaska Native, First Nations, Métis, and Inuit of Canada. The authors have identified best practices and lessons learned from collaborating with indigenous populations, presented in 2 categories: conceptual guidelines and health care delivery guidelines. Major themes include the importance of trust and communication, the delivery of culturally congruent health care, and the necessity of working in partnership with tribal entities for successful delivery of health care. Best practices in health care delivery with indigenous populations are presented.

The family health history (FHH) has long been used by nurses and other health care providers in clinical practice to determine if an individual, their family members, or their future generations are at an increased risk of heritable disease development. Information gleaned from the FHH can be used to better integrate preventive strategies into the plan of care. This report presents a summary of an exploratory pilot study that focused on the collection and use of FHH among a targeted group of Midwestern men and women. Findings suggest a need for efforts to further enhance the public's awareness of the importance of FHH.

This cross-sectional study examines health information–seeking behaviors and access to and use of technology among rural African Americans, Caucasians, and Hispanics. There was a low level of health information seeking across the sample. Few used smartphones or tablets and did not endorse receiving health information from their health care provider by e-mail. Printed materials remained a source of health information as did friends and family. Information should be shared using multiple platforms including more passive methods such as television and radio. More research is needed to ensure the health literacy, numeracy, and ability to navigate the online environment.

Costellia H. Talley and Karen Patricia Williams

This study examines the relationship between age, comorbidity, and breast and cervical cancer literacy in a sample of African American, Latina, and Arab women (N = 371) from Detroit, Michigan. The Age-adjusted Charlson Comorbidity Index (ACC) was used characterize the impact of age and comorbidity on breast and cervical cancer literacy. The relationship between ACC and breast and cervical cancer screening, and group differences, were assessed. There was a statistically significant difference between breast cancer literacy scores. ACC had a greater impact on breast cancer literacy for African Americans.

Felecia G. Wood, Elizabeth Alley, Spencer Baer, and Rebecca Johnson

A pilot program was initiated to improve self-management of type 2 diabetes by rural adults. Using an iOS-based, individually tailored pre-/postintervention to improve diabetes self-management, undergraduate students developed a native mobile application to help participants effectively manage their diabetes. Brief quizzes assessed diabetes knowledge. A diabetes dictionary and physical activity assessment provided additional support to users of the app. On completion of the pilot, data analysis indicated increased diabetes knowledge and self-efficacy, and ease of use of the technology. Native app technology permits ready access to important information for those living with type 2 diabetes.

Marilyn Cooper Handley and Daniel M. Avery Jr

This article reviews the persistent problem of smoking, especially as it relates to the rural and underserved population. The negative effects of smoking and disparities in health that occur as a result are highlighted. The article reviews the general state of smoking in the United States and discusses health-related issues and concerns of individuals who continue to smoke. The report explores individuals' rationale for smoking, barriers to cessation, and general knowledge related to the outcomes of smoking during pregnancy. The conclusions highlight the need for providers to provide information and interventions to reduce the smoking rates of pregnant women.

Michele Montgomery, Paige Johnson, and Patrick Ewell

This study identified risk factors (ie, high-risk racial/ethnic group, overweight/obesity, elevated blood pressure, elevated casual blood glucose, and the presence of acanthosis nigricans) for the development of type 2

NURSING CLINICS OF NORTH AMERICA

THE CLINICS ARE AVAILABLE ONLINE!
Access your subscription at:
www.theclinics.com

Foreword

Social Justice: A Basis for Health Care Delivery

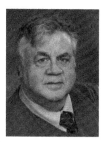

Stephen D. Krau, PhD, RN, CNE
Consulting Editor

With the passage of the Affordable Care Act, there was a concerted movement toward assuring that every citizen in the United States has access to affordable health care. This ideology has long been supported by other initiatives, including *Healthy People 2020.*[1] The extent to which this has come to fruition is difficult to capture due the variant terms used to describe underserved populations, or the context of health disparities, or defining geographical determinants. In some instances, defining disparities based on a particular populations or groups is not conveyed.[2] What is known is that the current health care system, despite this legislation and other initiatives, contains a disparity in health care coverage and countless treatment gaps for many citizens in the United States. The paramount desire to ensure that every citizen has access to affordable care has not occurred in the United States despite that every other country considered to have high income has such a system.[3]

The overriding concept that captures the issue of underserved population is portrayed in the definition of "health disparities," which in essence are the differences in groups where a particular group is socially disadvantaged. Braveman and colleagues identify that health care disparities are typically systematic, "plausibly avoidable health differences according to race/ethnicity, skin color, religion, or nationality; socioeconomic resources or position (reflected by, eg, income, wealth, education, or occupation); gender, sexual orientation, gender identity, age, geography, disability, illness, political or other affiliation; or other characteristics associated with discrimination or marginalization."[2] The notions of health disparity and equity are entrenched in social values and considerations and principles of ethics and human rights. Using ethical principles and beliefs, human rights, basic tenets of health disparities, and health care delivery would include those philosophical beliefs exemplified in **Box 1**.

Nurs Clin N Am 50 (2015) xiii–xv
http://dx.doi.org/10.1016/j.cnur.2015.07.002
0029-6465/15/$ – see front matter © 2015 Published by Elsevier Inc.

nursing.theclinics.com

> **Box 1**
> **Basic tenets addressing health disparities and health care equity**
>
> All people should be valued equally.
>
> Health has a particular value for individuals.
>
> Every person should be able to achieve his or her health status without regard to characteristics that have historically been linked to marginalization and/or discrimination.
>
> Health is of special importance to society.
>
> Accepted international standards of human rights obligate governments to promote and respect the human right to highest obtainable health.
>
> As suboptimal health can be an obstacle to overcoming social compromise and disadvantages, health differences unfavorably socially deprived groups are exceptionally objectionable.
>
> Resources crucial to health should be allocated fairly.
>
> Health equity is the expectation that underlies an obligation to reduce and finally eradicate health disparities.
>
> *Adapted from* Braveman P. Kumanyika S, Fielding J, et al. Health disparities and health equity: the issue is justice. Am J Public Health 2011;101(Suppl 1):S149–55.

It is unfeasible to describe health care equity and health care disparity without considering the notion of "social disadvantage."[2] Social disadvantage refers to those conditions some people systematically endure based on their relative status within a social hierarchy. This could be based on lack of political representation, low income, occupational rank, literacy level, or education. Health disparities or inequities impact disadvantaged groups by actually putting them at higher risk for disadvantage. This results in creating situations where overcoming the social disadvantage can be more difficult. Even though this conundrum is clear, causality cannot be demonstrated or proven. Causality is often a major focus but should not displace the outcome, which is inadequate health care accessibility or affordability for many individuals.

One perspective that addresses disparities through a systematic approach involves the contemplation of social justice. Justice is one of the four key medical ethical principles. It is probably lesser known than the principles of "autonomy" (self-determination), "nonmaleficence" (do no wrong), or the principle of "beneficence" (do the right thing).[4] Within the health care system, "justice" can be considered that persons with the same medical conditions should have availability of the same treatment options. "Social justice" refers to a distribution of goods or services within a societal context. It focuses on the persons or groups that influence the distribution of services or merchandise. This includes health care treatment accessibility and availability.

Social justice provides the basis for action from all health care providers as catalysts to social change. Clearly there are barriers many health care providers face in this role. Logically, for nurses and physicians there can be a sense that legislative policies and political influences pose insurmountable obstacles for social change. With other influential decision-makers, whose focus might not be grounded in social justice, nurses and physicians can experience a sense of disempowerment, disillusionment, and futility. However, nurses and doctors are socially postured to exert more influence than the disadvantaged patients and groups they serve. Ethical principles and human rights demand focused attention and care on those facing extreme obstacles. These principles can protect many people and groups from serious challenges and threats, not the least of which is the disparity in health care.

Stephen D. Krau, PhD, RN, CNE
Vanderbilt University Medical Center
309 Godchaux Hall, 461 21st Avenue South
Nashville, TN 37240, USA

E-mail address:
steve.krau@vanderbilt.edu

REFERENCES

1. U.S. Department of Health and Human Services Office of Disease Prevention and Health Promotion. Healthy People 2020. November 2010. Available at: http://www. healthypeople.gov/. Accessed July 7, 2015.
2. Braveman P, Kumanyika S, Fielding J, et al. Health disparities and health equity: the issue is justice. Am J Public Health 2011;101(Suppl 1):S149–55.
3. List J. Beyond charity—social justice and health care. Virtual Mentor 2011;13(8): 565–8.
4. Freeman J. Health medicine and justice: designing a fair and equitable health care system. Friday Harbor (WA): Copernicus Healthcare; 2015.

Preface

Rural and Other Medically Underserved Populations

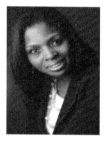
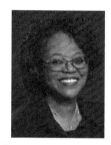

JoAnn S. Oliver, PhD, RN, CNE   Sandra Millon Underwood, PhD, RN, FAAN
Editors

Millions of Americans are characterized as medically underserved given that they live in a *medically underserved area* with little or no health care or that they are part of a *medically underserved group or population* known to experience economic, cultural, or linguistic barriers to health care.[1,2] Rural and urban dwellers, low-income groups, racial and ethnic minorities, children, older adults, and individuals with special health care needs are characterized as priority populations by the National Center for Health Statistics and the Agency for Health Care Research and Quality given that they face myriad economic, social, cultural, geographic, and systemic barriers to health care access, health care delivery, and health care utilization.[3]

Nurses are highly regarded in the health care community. Likewise, given the scope of their knowledge, the breadth of their practice, and the depth of their commitment to care for all who are in need, they have been noted to be a critical lever for change relative to addressing the needs of these and other disparate groups and populations. Our understanding of the needs and concerns of rural and medically underserved populations and our experiences working in rural and other medically underserved areas, along with those of our collaborating authors, served as the impetus for this special issue of *Nursing Clinics of North America*.

This issue highlights the work of an esteemed group of nurse clinicians, educators, and researchers whose clinical practices, research, and programs of scholarship are dedicated to improving the health condition of rural and underserved populations. Included among the work cited are reports that address hearing loss of adults with type 2 diabetes, the clinical implications of food insecurity among underserved populations; barriers to smoking cessation in rural and underserved pregnant women, best practices for establishing partnerships with indigenous populations of North America, the integration of family health history in primary care practice, the nonemergency use of emergency medical services among rural populations, and the use of mobile devices to access information in rural a setting. We believe that insights gleaned from these

Nurs Clin N Am 50 (2015) xvii–xviii
http://dx.doi.org/10.1016/j.cnur.2015.07.001
0029-6465/15/$ – see front matter © 2015 Published by Elsevier Inc.

nursing.theclinics.com

reports, along with the others included in this special issue, will collectively provide nurse clinicians, educators, researchers, and consumers alike a unique perspective on an array of health care concerns and conditions faced by rural, urban, low-income, racial, and ethnic minority population groups, children and older adults, and persons with chronic health conditions. As a result, it is believed that insights shared and gleaned from these authors will positively impact nursing practice and will result in improved patient outcomes.

JoAnn S. Oliver, PhD, RN, CNE
Associate Professor, The University of Alabama
Capstone College of Nursing
Tuscaloosa, AL 35401, USA

Sandra Millon Underwood, PhD, RN, FAAN
Professor, University of Wisconsin Milwaukee
College of Nursing
1921 Easr Hartford, Milwaukee
WI 53211, USA

E-mail addresses:
joliver@ua.edu (J.S. Oliver)
underwoo@uwm.edu (S.M. Underwood)

REFERENCES

1. National Center for Health Statistics. Health, United States, 2014: with special feature on adults aged 55–64. Hyattsville (MD); Washington, DC: US Government Printing Office; 2015.
2. DC.gov. Medically underserved areas—populations. 2015. Available at: http://doh.dc.gov/service/medically-underserved-areas-populations. Accessed May 28, 2015.
3. Priority Populations. Agency for Healthcare Research and Quality, Rockville (MD). 2015. Available at: http://www.ahrq.gov/health-care-information/priority-populations/index.html. Accessed May 28, 2015.

Diabetes and Hearing Loss Among Underserved Populations

Donna Calvin, PhD, FNP-BC[a],*, Sanreka R. Watley, MS[b]

KEYWORDS

- Diabetes • Hearing loss • Microvascular circulation • Microvascular complications
- Minorities • Underserved populations • Consequences of hearing loss

KEY POINTS

- Diabetes affects the vasculature of the middle ear, resulting in hearing loss.
- Early detection and treatment can help prevent the complications associated with hearing loss.
- There are strategies and devices that can help alleviate the complications of hearing loss.

INTRODUCTION

Type 2 diabetes (T2DM) and its resulting complications exact a devastating personal, social, and economic burden on the United States population. Since 1980, the prevalence of diabetes in the United States has more than tripled. Approximately 29.1 million people, or 9.3% of the United States population, are living with diabetes, and 8.1 million of these people remain undiagnosed.[1] Alarmingly, 86 million people are estimated to have prediabetes, a condition whereby blood glucose levels are higher than normal but not at a diagnostic level for diabetes.[1] The presence of prediabetes increases one's risk of developing diabetes.

Minority populations disproportionately bear the burden of T2DM. Compared with white Americans whose rate of T2DM is 7.6%, Native Americans (15.9%), African Americans (13.2%), and Hispanics (12.8%) are approximately twice as likely to develop the disease.[1]

These populations are also more apt to develop the devastating microvascular complications of T2DM, namely blindness, lower limb amputation, and kidney failure.[2] Low socioeconomic status (SES) and substandard environmental conditions are often associated with poor health outcomes, resulting in higher risks of microvascular and

Disclosures: None.
[a] Department of Nursing, Governors State University, 1 University Parkway, University Park, IL 60484, USA; [b] Unitron, Northern California, HI, USA
* Corresponding author. 20210 Saint Andrews Court, Olympia Fields, IL 60461.
E-mail address: dcalvin@govst.edu

Nurs Clin N Am 50 (2015) 449–456
http://dx.doi.org/10.1016/j.cnur.2015.05.001
0029-6465/15/$ – see front matter © 2015 Elsevier Inc. All rights reserved.

microvascular complications. The disparities have often been attributed to the fact that persons with T2DM who are of low SES do not receive optimal health care, and often the environment does not support their ability to adequately manage the disease.[3–6] Minorities are also disproportionately represented in the lower SES category.

DIABETES AND HEARING LOSS

Data from the National Health and Nutrition Examination Survey (NHANES) suggest that among persons with diabetes between the ages of 50 and 69 years, more than 70% have high-frequency hearing loss and one-third also have low-frequency or mid-frequency hearing loss. Hearing loss is approximately twice as common in adults with diabetes as in those who do not have the disease. The link between diabetes and hearing loss is evident across all frequencies.[7–9]

The prevalence of hearing loss among older adults with or without T2DM is significant. Hearing loss is listed as the third most prevalent chronic illness among the elderly population; 36 million people report having hearing loss. It is estimated that 25% to 40% of the United States population aged 65 years or older has some degree of hearing loss. This prevalence rises with age.[10,11] Hearing impairment may be due to a problem with conduction, the sensorineural pathway, or both. Presbycusis is a progressive sensorineural problem that makes one less able to hear high-pitched tones and filter background noise, and is the most common reason for hearing loss. Presbycusis is age related and starts around 50 years of age.[12] Persons with T2DM are twice as likely as those without T2DM to have a greater prevalence of hearing loss.[7,9,13] Research has shown that White males and females with T2DM have a greater prevalence of hearing loss than minorities.[7,9,14] However, there is a dearth of information concerning the ethnic-related differences in rates among individuals with diabetes and hearing loss. As already stated, minorities and persons of low SES in general do not receive optimal health care, including screening for hearing loss. Therefore, the true prevalence of the disease among the underserved population is not known. As the underserved population is disproportionately affected by the well-known microvascular complications caused by T2DM, there exists the potential for hearing loss also to disproportionately affect this population. The NHANES data also indicated that those who are of lower SES and have lower levels of education have a higher prevalence of T2DM hearing loss (**Table 1**).[9]

Other well-known causes of hearing loss should be ruled out to ensure that one receives optimal care[12]:

- Ear wax: conductive hearing loss
- Otosclerosis of the malleus, incus, and stapes bones
- Infections such as meningitis, mumps, and measles
- Neurologic disorders such as multiple sclerosis
- Acoustic neuroma
- Ménière disease
- Damage to the cochlea or the eighth nerve producing sensorineural loss from head trauma
- Effects of ototoxic medications (eg, aminoglycoside antibiotics, diuretics, salicylates, and antineoplastic agents)
- Noise-induced hearing loss

WHAT IS HEARING LOSS?

The softest sounds a person with normal hearing can hear is 25 dB or lower. When one is unable to hear at this level, signs and symptoms of hearing loss become apparent.

Table 1
Prevalence of high-frequency hearing loss of mild or greater severity

	No. of Participants with Diabetes (N = 399)	Prevalence of Hearing Loss (%)	No. of Participants Without Diabetes (N = 4741)	Prevalence of Hearing Loss
Age (y)				
20–49	97	44.2	3232	18.6
50–59	111	70.5	727	55.7
60–69	191	89.9	782	77.7
Race/ethnicity				
Non-Hispanic white	139	72.8	2311	34.8
Non-Hispanic black	97	46.9	956	19.7
Mexican American	118	53.3	1090	22.3
Other	45	74.5	384	25.0
Income-poverty ratio				
≤1.0	88	67.9	796	26.1
>1.0	273	67.9	3535	31.6

Data from Bainbridge KE, Hoffman HJ, Cowie CC. Diabetes and hearing impairment in the United States: audiometric evidence from the National Health and Nutrition Examination Survey, 1999 to 2004. Ann Intern Med 2008;149(1):1–10.

However, the person with hearing loss may not recognize a deficit. The spouse or caregiver will often report that the patient: turns up the volume on the TV; has difficulty talking over the telephone or having a conversation in a noisy environment; often states "speak louder," "I can't hear you," "why are you mumbling"; cups the hand over the ear during normal conversations or gets closer to the person; and often gives inappropriate responses or misinterprets what has been said.

See **Table 2** for classification of hearing loss.[12,15]

PATHOPHYSIOLOGY OF TYPE 2 DIABETES MICROVASCULAR DISEASE AND HEARING LOSS

Retinopathies that lead to blindness, neuropathy that may result in one having a lower extremity amputation, and chronic kidney disease that may progress to kidney failure, are all well-known microvascular diseases associated with T2DM. T2DM seems to

Table 2
Classification of hearing loss

Degree of Hearing Loss	Hearing Loss Range (dB HL)
Normal	≤25
Mild	26–40
Moderate	41–55
Moderately severe	56–70
Severe	71–90
Profound	≥91

Data from Wallhagen MI, Pettengill E, Whiteside M. Sensory impairment in older adults: PART 1: hearing loss. Am J Nurs 2006;106(10):40–8.

similarly affect the vasculature and neural system of the inner ear, which often leads to hearing loss.[8,16,17] T2DM leads to hyperviscosity (ie, thick sludgy blood) which contributes to vascular complications. Abnormally high levels of plasma glucose primarily affect red blood cells and the vascular endothelial cells, including the walls of capillaries. In T2DM, elevated blood viscosity plays a major role in the development of microvascular diseases by altering microcirculation and leading to insufficient tissue perfusion. Red cells must be able to freely pass through the capillaries to supply oxygen to the surrounding tissues.[18–20]

In T2DM hearing loss it is reasonable to consider that hyperviscosity attributable to high blood glucose levels cause tiny blood vessels in the inner ear to break, disrupting sound reception. This process also disrupts the microcirculation in the vestibular portion of the inner ear (cochlea) by injuring or clogging the tiny blood vessels that nourish the vestibular end organs (hair cells and nerves).[16,17] Persons with diabetes often have less keratin, a protein that lines the ear canal, which also contributes to hearing loss.[7,16,18] Consequently, individuals with T2DM are twice as likely as those without T2DM to have hearing loss.[7]

THE PHYSICAL, EMOTIONAL, AND SOCIAL IMPACT OF HEARING LOSS

Hearing loss is associated with a variety of physical, emotional, and social problems. Persons with hearing loss have poorer health outcomes and are less likely to engage in healthy behaviors than those with good hearing.[11,21,22] More importantly, their quality of life is often severely compromised. The inability to effectively communicate leads to frustration, sadness, and depression. Often they suffer from anxiety and paranoia, become less active in the community, and isolate themselves from others. Such individuals may not be able to continue to drive because they are distracted by background noise such as a horn blowing or railroad warnings; they have difficulty hearing high-pitched sounds such as that of a siren from an emergency vehicle, and thus are unable to respond in a timely manner. Hearing loss may also lead to an inability to continue employment, thus decreasing one's income.[12,21]

In addition to the aforementioned complications directly related to hearing loss, the vestibular portion of the ear is often damaged, leading to serious alterations in motor skills that can lead to an increased incidence of falls. Some of the most prominent signs of vestibular damage include: difficulty walking straight or turning corners, and difficulty with coordination; inability to maintain straight posture as a result of looking down to confirm the location of the ground; and a greater tendency to touch or hold something (eg, wall, railing) when standing.[12,23]

PREVENTING PROGRESSION OF HEARING LOSS

Hearing loss caused by T2DM, like most of the microvascular complications of diabetes, may be preventable. All are due in some part to aging and impaired microcirculatory blood flow. It is evident that basic lifestyle changes, specifically increased physical activity, improves microcirculation. One cannot do anything about aging, but maintaining a healthy diet, controlling blood glucose and blood pressure, and increasing physical activity may help to prevent the occurrence and progression of all diabetes complications including hearing loss.[24–27]

IMPLICATIONS FOR HEALTH CARE PROVIDERS

Early identification and treatment is crucial in ameliorating the negative consequences of hearing loss. Hearing impairment results in a significant physical, emotional, social, and financial burden on the individual in addition to a great financial burden on the health care system. One of the goals of Healthy People 2020 is to reduce the prevalence and severity of disorders of hearing and balance, with the objective of improving the rate of screening for hearing loss.[28] The most recent data reveal that less than 29% of adults aged 20 to 69, compared with 40.6% among those aged 70 and older, underwent a hearing examination in the past 5 years. There is a definite need to improve the rates of screening, especially in the 20- to 69-year age group, because the greatest difference in the prevalence of hearing loss between persons with T2DM and those without is soon among the younger population.[9,29]

Standards of care guidelines for T2DM include routine screening for eye disease, nerve damage, kidney disease, cardiovascular disease, gum disease, lower extremity complications, and depression. Many organizations including the American Academy of Family Physicians and The American Geriatric Society do not include screening for hearing loss in the guidelines for managing T2DM. Although the American Diabetes Association recognizes the link between diabetes and hearing loss, the 2015 Standards of Medical Care in Diabetes also does not include routine screening for hearing loss.[30]

Routine screening can be done in the office of the primary care provider. It can and should be included in the routine preparation for one to see the provider along with vital signs. Medicare reimburses primary care providers for a one-time preventive screening for hearing loss.[31,32] There are several hand-held devices that can be used to screen for hearing loss, in the physician's office, in less than 5 minutes. There are various written and computerized self-screening tools that can be used at home, the results of which can be discussed with one's provider.[12,33]

Once patients are identified as having some degree of hearing loss they should be referred to an ear/nose/throat physician, audiologist, or hearing instrument specialist for further testing and to determine which affordable device will best meet their needs. Medicare will reimburse the provider for testing but does not pay for hearing aids.[31,32] Many treatment options are available for patients with hearing loss, such as hearing aids, telephone-amplifying devices, captioned telephones, louder door bells, or bells that do not use high-frequency tones.[12,34] There are also listening training programs that help improve one's ability to function with the hearing deficit.[35]

Hearing aids are the best solution for those with moderate to severe hearing loss. However, for some, especially the elderly underserved population, they may be inaccessible. Hearing aids can be expensive, ranging from a few hundred dollars to a few thousand. The average cost of a quality well-fitted device is approximately $4400.[36] Despite the proven social and physical benefits of improving one's ability to hear, Medicare currently does not pay for hearing aids, although in most states Medicaid will pay for them.[33]

Many hearing aid companies have programs that lend assistance in helping clients obtain hearing devices. Other sources of assistance include the Veterans Administration, Hear Now, and organizations such as the Lions Clubs, Rotary Clubs, and United Way (**Table 3**).[35]

IMPLICATIONS FOR NURSING

Although there may be access to hearing devices, many persons with hearing loss remain undiagnosed and thus are never referred to a hearing specialist. Many of the programs previously mentioned have income guidelines, and some Medicare recipients may not fall within the range of income to qualify for the programs.

Nurses are at the forefront of providing health promotion and prevention.

Table 3 Resources for self-screening and care		
Organization	**Resource**	**URL**
Better Hearing Institute	Self-administered written and auditory hearing screenings Several brochures discussing various topics related to hearing loss	http://www.betterhearing.org/check-your-hearing http://www.betterhearing.org/hearingpedia/bhi-archives/eguides
Hearing Loss Association of America	Overview of hearing loss, list of assistive devices including hearing aids Listening training programs Resources for financial support	http://hearingloss.org/content/understanding-hearing-loss http://hearingloss.org/content/financial-assistance-programs-foundations
American Speech-Language-Hearing Association	Overview of communication disorders, resources for services Self-administered written screening	http://www.asha.org/public/ http://www.asha.org/public/hearing/Self-Test-for-Hearing-Loss/

Nurses can and should:

- Ensure that all patients, including those who are at risk of being underserved, are aware of the link between diabetes and hearing loss
- Raise awareness among health care providers and promote screening for hearing loss in the community
- Advocate for access to affordable care and assistive devices
- Advocate for all payers, including Medicare, to fund hearing devices for the hearing impaired
- Develop research projects to help determine the impact of hearing loss among the underserved populations with T2DM

SUMMARY

The prevalence of diabetes complications among minorities and underserved populations is increasing. In general, there has been negligible improvement in controlling T2DM and its complications. Hearing loss seems to be a hidden complication of T2DM. There is a lack of published information concerning the association between diabetes and hearing loss. Most of the information is found within the audiological world. Providers, specifically primary care providers, need to be aware of this association. The impact of hearing loss on the individual can be devastating. Persons without T2DM and with hearing loss have a higher rate of hospitalization and mortality.[22,37] Thus, it is safe to say that those with T2DM and hearing loss are even more vulnerable to health problems. Further study is required to truly understand the impact of hearing loss on minorities and underserved populations with T2DM. Most importantly, nurses and providers must ensure that persons with T2DM are afforded screening and treatment for hearing loss. Hearing is not a luxury but a necessity.

ACKNOWLEDGMENTS

We would like to thank Paul Blobaum, MA, MS, Scholarly Communications Librarian Governors State University.

REFERENCES

1. American Diabetes Association. Statistics about diabetes. 2014. Available at: http://www.diabetes.org/diabetes-basics/statistics/?loc=superfooter. Accessed January 4, 2015.
2. American Diabetes Association. Health disparities. 2014. Available at: http://www.diabetes.org/advocacy/advocacy-priorities/health-disparities.html. Accessed December 28, 2014.
3. Atherton K, Power C. Health inequalities with the national statistics-socioeconomic classification: disease risk factors and health in the 1958 British birth cohort. Eur J Public Health 2007;17(5):486–91.
4. Grintsova O, Maier W, Mielck A. Inequalities in health care among patients with type 2 diabetes by individual socio-economic status (SES) and regional deprivation: a systematic literature review. Int J Equity Health 2014;13(1):43.
5. Raphael D. Poverty in childhood and adverse health outcomes in adulthood. Maturitas 2011;69(1):22–6.
6. Ricci-Cabello I, Ruiz-Pérez I, Labry-Lima D, et al. Do social inequalities exist in terms of the prevention, diagnosis, treatment, control and monitoring of diabetes? A systematic review. Health Soc Care Community 2010;18(6):572–87.
7. Bainbridge KE, Hoffman HJ, Cowie CC. Diabetes and hearing impairment in the United States: audiometric evidence from the National Health and Nutrition Examination Survey, 1999 to 2004. Ann Intern Med 2008;149(1):1–10.
8. Ren J, Zhao P, Chen L, et al. Hearing loss in middle-aged subjects with type 2 diabetes mellitus. Arch Med Res 2009;40(1):18–23.
9. Bainbridge KE, Hoffman HJ, Cowie CC. Risk factors for hearing impairment among U.S. adults with diabetes: National Health and Nutrition Examination Survey 1999-2004. Diabetes Care 2011;34(7):1540–5.
10. Helzner EP, Cauley JA, Pratt SR, et al. Race and sex differences in age-related hearing loss: the health, aging and body composition study. J Am Geriatr Soc 2005;53(12):2119–27.
11. Lin FR, Metter EJ, O'Brien RJ, et al. Hearing loss and incident dementia. Arch Neurol 2011;68(2):214–20.
12. American Speech-Language-Hearing Association. Hearing loss. Available at: http://www.asha.org/public/hearing/Hearing-Loss/. Accessed January 6, 2015.
13. Lerman-Garber I, Cuevas-Ramos D, Valdés S, et al. Sensorineural hearing loss-A common finding in early-onset type 2 diabetes mellitus. Endocr Pract 2012;18(4): 549–57.
14. Akinpelu OV, Mujica-Mota M, Daniel SJ. Is type 2 diabetes mellitus associated with alterations in hearing? A systematic review and meta-analysis. Laryngoscope 2014;124(3):767–76.
15. Wallhagen MI, Pettengill E, Whiteside M. Sensory impairment in older adults: PART 1: hearing loss. Am J Nurs 2006;106(10):40–8.
16. Lisowska G, Namyslowski G, Morawski K, et al. Cochlear dysfunction and diabetic microangiopathy. Scand Audiol 2001;30(1):199–203.
17. Fukushima H, Cureoglu S, Schachern PA, et al. Effects of type 2 diabetes mellitus on cochlear structure in humans. Arch Otolaryngol Head Neck Surg 2006;132(9): 934–8.
18. Cho YI, Mooney MP, Cho DJ. Hemorheological disorders in diabetes mellitus. J Diabetes Sci Technol 2008;2(6):1130–8.
19. Grant P. Diabetes mellitus as a prothrombotic condition. J Intern Med 2007; 262(2):157–72.

20. Reid HL, Vigilance J, Wright-Pascoe RA, et al. The influence of persistent hyperglycaemia on hyperfibrinogenaemia and hyperviscosity in diabetes mellitus. West Indian Med J 2000;49(4):281–4.
21. Ciorba A, Bianchini C, Pelucchi S, et al. The impact of hearing loss on the quality of life of elderly adults. Clin Interv Aging 2012;7:159–63.
22. Genther DJ, Frick KD, Chen D, et al. Association of hearing loss with hospitalization and burden of disease in older adults. JAMA 2013;309(22):2322–4.
23. Vestibular Disorders Association. Symptoms of vestibular disorders. Available at: http://vestibular.org/understanding-vestibular-disorder/symptoms#other. Accessed January 5, 2015.
24. Klonizakis M, Winter E. Effects of arm-cranking exercise in cutaneous microcirculation in older, sedentary people. Microvasc Res 2011;81(3):331–6.
25. Gerovasili V, Drakos S, Kravari M, et al. Physical exercise improves the peripheral microcirculation of patients with chronic heart failure. J Cardiopulm Rehabil Prev 2009;29(6):385–91.
26. Khavandi K, Brownrigg J, Hankir M, et al. Interrupting the natural history of diabetes mellitus: lifestyle, pharmacological and surgical strategies targeting disease progression. Curr Vasc Pharmacol 2014;12(1):155–67.
27. Colberg SR, Sigal RJ, Fernhall B, et al. Exercise and type 2 diabetes: the American College of Sports Medicine and the American Diabetes Association: joint position statement. Diabetes Care 2010;33(12):e147–67.
28. U.S. Department of Health and Human Services. Healthy people. 2020. Available at: http://www.healthypeople.gov/2020/topics-objectives/topic/hearing-and-other-sensory-or-communication-disorders/objectives. Assessed February 12, 2015.
29. Konrad-Martin D, Reavis KM, Austin D, et al. Hearing impairment in relation to severity of diabetes in a veteran cohort. Ear Hear 2015. http://dx.doi.org/10.1097/AUD.0000000000000137.
30. American Diabetes Association. Standards of medical care in diabetes—2015. Diabetes Care 2015;38(Suppl. 1):S1–SXXX.
31. Donahue A, Dubno JR, Beck L. Guest editorial: accessible and affordable hearing health care for adults with mild to moderate hearing loss. Ear Hear 2010; 31(1):2–6.
32. Johnson CE, Danhauer JL, Koch LL, et al. Hearing and balance screening and referrals for Medicare patients: a national survey of primary care physicians. J Am Acad Audiol 2008;19(2):171–90.
33. Better Hearing Institute. Guide to financial assistance for hearing aids. Available at: http://www.betterhearing.org/sites/default/files/hearingpedia-resources/Financial_Assistance_for_Hearing_Aids.pdf. Accessed February 12, 2015.
34. Hearing Loss Association of America. Hearing assistive technology. Available at: http://hearingloss.org/content/hearing-assistive-technology. Accessed February 12, 2015.
35. Hearing Loss Association of America. Listening training programs. Available at: http://hearingloss.org/content/listening-training-programs. Accessed February 12, 2015.
36. Cropp I, AARP. Why do hearing aids cost so much? 2014. Available at: http://www.aarp.org/health/conditions-treatments/info-05-2011/hearing-aids-cost.html. Accessed January 19, 2015.
37. Genther DJ, Betz J, Pratt S, et al. Association of hearing impairment and mortality in older adults. J Gerontol A Biol Sci Med Sci 2015;70(1):85–90.

Cardiovascular Health Among an Underserved Population: Clinical Implications

Margaret T. Bowers, DNP, RN, FNP-BC

KEYWORDS

- Cardiovascular health • Underserved population • Disparities
- Treatment adherence • Cardiovascular disease

KEY POINTS

- Cardiovascular disease remains the primary cause of morbidity and mortality in the United States.
- The recent focus of cardiovascular care has shifted from treatment of disease to promotion of health.
- Identification of those at high risk for poor cardiovascular health in adulthood should begin during early adolescence.
- Disparities in cardiovascular disease are more prevalent in the underserved population.

INTRODUCTION

Cardiovascular disease remains the primary cause of morbidity and mortality in the United States despite the reduction in strokes and coronary heart disease over the previous decade.[1] Historically, clinical practice guidelines have focused on treatment rather than prevention of diseases such as hypertension, coronary artery disease, and hyperlipidemia. Recently, these clinical practice guidelines have included comorbid conditions as significant factors to be considered in managing these disease states.[2] Despite efforts at treatment of these conditions, disparities in cardiovascular care remain prevalent in underserved populations.[2–4]

Risk assessment, disease prevention, and improvement in cardiovascular health comprise the current focus of the 2013 cardiovascular joint clinical practice guidelines from the American College of Cardiology/American Heart Association (ACC/AHA).[5] Parallel implementation of both prevention and treatment guidelines in addition to clinical practice recommendations for management of hypertension, coronary artery

Disclosures: None.
Duke University School of Nursing, 3322 Duke University, Durham, NC 27710, USA
E-mail address: Margaret.bowers@duke.edu

Nurs Clin N Am 50 (2015) 457–464
http://dx.doi.org/10.1016/j.cnur.2015.05.002
0029-6465/15/$ – see front matter © 2015 Elsevier Inc. All rights reserved.

disease, and hyperlipidemia provide a dual-pronged approach to improving cardiovascular health and reducing chronic cardiovascular diseases.

CARDIOVASCULAR HEALTH

The ACC/AHA defines cardiovascular health as poor, intermediate, or ideal based on set criteria for 7 metrics, which include both risk factors and behaviors.[6] The 7 metrics include risk factors such as elevated total cholesterol, blood pressure, and fasting blood glucose, and behaviors such as smoking status, eating a healthy diet, engaging in sufficient physical activity, and maintaining normal body weight.[7] Ideal cardiovascular health exists when there is no evidence of cardiovascular disease while meeting the ideal criteria across each of these 7 health metrics.[6] The focus on health promotion and disease prevention means that there is potential to reduce morbidity and mortality across race and gender. According to the AHA, the impact goals for 2020 are to focus on improving these 7 health metrics of cardiovascular health and to reduce cardiovascular disease and stroke by 20%. Identification of those at high risk for poor cardiovascular health in adulthood should begin during early adolescence (**Box 1**).[7]

In the United States, children aged 12 to 19 years have variable risk for poor cardiovascular health based on data from the National Health and Nutrition Examination Survey (NHANES) in 2012 and diet data from 2009 to 2011. The health behaviors that provide the most significant opportunity for improvement include a healthy diet, adequate physical activity, and reduction in body weight. Reduction in smoking has demonstrated a dramatic improvement in the adolescent population, with 87.1% non-smokers and 12.9% smokers. There remains an opportunity to focus on smoking cessation as smoking is associated with poor health outcomes, many of which are avoidable.[5,6]

In addition to improvement of health behaviors, focusing on improvement of the risk factors for the development of cardiovascular disease must be addressed. Although the data from the NHANES study suggest that both blood pressure and fasting plasma glucose levels achieved the ideal metric for cardiovascular health in the adolescent population, these risk factors must continue to meet the metrics into adulthood and across diverse populations. Through achievement of meeting targets of healthy behavior and risk factors, the focus of cardiovascular care can be shifted to secondary prevention rather than treatment of acute cardiovascular conditions such as acute myocardial infarction and stroke. Population-level risk reduction and improvement in cardiovascular health can be achieved with modest movement from poor to both intermediate and ideal categories of the 7 health metrics.[5,6] Based on these data, there are opportunities to improve physical activity and diet in 12- to 19-year-olds

Box 1	
Seven metrics of cardiovascular health	
Factors	**Behaviors**
Optimal total cholesterol	Not smoking
Optimal blood pressure	Healthy diet pattern
Optimal fasting blood glucose	Sufficient physical activity
—	Appropriate energy balance evidenced by normal body weight

Adapted from Mozaffarian D, Benjamin EJ, Go AS. Heart disease and stroke statistics—2015 update. Circulation 2015;131:e40.

and continue the successful efforts at smoking cessation and blood pressure control. Focusing on cardiovascular health in this age group has implications for improving health in the over-twenties population, with downstream reduction in cardiovascular morbidity and mortality.

Looking at individuals in the 20- to 49-year age group and the over-50s age range within the NHANES data, there are similarities among areas for improvement across the board, including enhancing a healthy diet. Across the all of these age ranges (12–50+), the data did not reveal any age group achieving greater than 1% prevalence for a healthy diet. As a nation struggling with the increase in obesity, the prevalence of ideal body mass index (BMI), 34.6% in ages 20 to 49 years and 26.7% in those older than 50, suggests that current strategies for increasing physical activity and following a healthy diet have fallen short. Addressing strategies for improving dietary and BMI cardiovascular health metrics are challenging in isolation because of the multiple factors that influence success. Beyond weight and BMI, measurement the indirect measures of optimal fasting blood glucose and optimal total cholesterol provide quantitative measures with which to evaluate success in these metrics.

CARDIOVASCULAR DISEASE

In the United States the incidence of hypertension, coronary heart disease, and stroke are diverse across both age and gender. The difference in cardiovascular mortality across race and gender remains significant, with the highest risk among black males and the lowest among white females (**Table 1**).[8] Factors contributing to this high mortality include elevated levels of blood glucose, blood pressure, and cholesterol, increasing the risk of myocardial infarction, stroke, heart failure, renal disease, and peripheral vascular disease. Black females have a higher prevalence of hypertension than black males and, compared with whites, 9% to 17% higher prevalence males than in females. The prevalence of coronary heart disease is highest in white males, followed by black males, black females, and white females. Stroke prevalence is similar across both genders, and race data was not reported. Targeting cardiovascular prevention and treatments at the populations at highest overall mortality risk, such as black men, can narrow the gap of cardiovascular disease across race and gender.

There are a growing number of Hispanic Americans from multiethnic origins who represent one of the most rapidly increasing ethnicities in the United States, and it

Table 1
Prevalence of hypertension, coronary heart disease, and stroke by gender and race of United States adults

	Male	Female
Hypertension	42.6% Black	47.0% Black
	33.4% White	30.7% White
Coronary heart disease	7.8% Overall	4.6% Overall
	7.3% Black	5.9% Black
	7.7% White	4.2% White
Stroke	2.7% Overall	2.6% Overall

Data from Mozaffarian D, Benjamin EJ, Go AS. Heart disease and stroke statistics—2015 update. Circulation 2015;131:e29322; with permission; and Centers for Disease Control and Prevention (CDC). Prevalence of coronary heart disease; United States, 2006–2010. MMWR Morb Mortal Wkly Rep 2011;60(40):1377–81. Available at: http://www.cdc.gov/mmwr/preview/mmwrhtml/mm6040a1.htm#tab1.

is anticipated that by 2050 they will represent one-third of the population.[9] As the Hispanic population increases, so will the prevalence of diseases linked to chronic illnesses such as diabetes, uncontrolled hypertension, dyslipidemia, and obesity.[10] Data analysis of the cardiovascular risk among the Hispanic population is challenging owing to the fact that multiethnic data are frequently unreported and are focused on only one ethnicity, such as Mexican Americans. The AHA identifies the Mexican American population at risk by both race and gender, as noted in **Table 2**. According to the Study of Latinos/Hispanic Community Health Study, a comprehensive evaluation sponsored by the National Heart, Lung and Blood Institute looking at the prevalence of chronic disease focused on Hispanics and Latinos, there is a 16.9% prevalence of diagnosed and undiagnosed diabetes mellitus across both genders.[11] By focusing on prevention of these chronic health conditions in a growing Hispanic population, there is a chance to mitigate the adverse consequences and improve overall health through reducing the incidence of cardiovascular disease, diabetes, hypertension, dyslipidemia, and obesity.

UNDERSERVED POPULATIONS

Underserved populations are those in which there is social marginalization as a result of limited income and literacy, resource-poor communities, racial/ethnic minority status, or recent migration to the United States.[4] Within these underserved populations, the lack of community-based resources such as safe environments in which to exercise and options for healthy food choices has an impact on cardiovascular health. Limited access to nutritious food and increased access to fast food with high sodium and fat content have a direct effect on the development of hypertension, diabetes, elevated cholesterol, and obesity, and generally places individuals at increased risk for cardiovascular disease. Leading a sedentary lifestyle is another health behavior that affects effective treatment of hypertension, diabetes, elevated cholesterol, and obesity.

In a systematic review by Walton-Moss and colleagues[12] evaluating community-based interventions targeted at improving cardiovascular health in vulnerable populations, the investigators cited variable definitions of vulnerable populations as posing a challenge in evaluating studies. Despite these diverse definitions, vulnerable and underserved populations are at higher risk for the development of chronic cardiovascular diseases (see earlier discussion).

Evidence-based guidelines are available for many chronic cardiovascular diseases such as hypertension, hyperlipidemia, and coronary artery disease, which are prevalent in underserved populations. Implementation of these guidelines should be considered as a strategy to improve cardiovascular health. However, adherence to these

Table 2 Prevalence of disease among Mexican Americans in the United States		
	Male (%)	Female (%)
Cardiovascular disease	33.4	30.7
Elevated cholesterol	48.1	44.7
Hypertension	30.1	28.8

Data from Go AS, Mozaffarian D, Roger VL, et al; on behalf of the American Heart Association Statistics Committee and Stroke Statistics Subcommittee. Heart disease and stroke statistics—2013 update: a report from the American Heart Association. Circulation 2013;127:e6–24.

therapies is affected by cost, availability of treatments (including pharmaceuticals), and access to care. Lowest adherence to cardiovascular medications is highest among marginalized groups.[13,14]

In a Canadian study looking at cultural barriers to participation in cardiac rehabilitation programs, Savage and colleagues[15] identified that although there is universal health care, there is a 5.4-year difference in life expectancy of men of lower socioeconomic status compared with men of highest socioeconomic status, with an 8.4-year difference in women in the same comparison groups. The investigators concluded that participation in cardiac rehabilitation and making healthy lifestyle choices are socially sensitive matters.[15]

Because socioeconomic status is such a key determinant of health status, it must be addressed in the context of improving cardiovascular health. There are many barriers to deal with in an underserved population that make it challenging to achieve the previously identified cardiovascular metrics. Commonly identified barriers include:

- Easy access to local fast food and convenience stores
- Limited access to fresh fruits or vegetables and the high cost of these items
- Access to safe walking/exercise environment, parks, or gym facilities
- Multiple role demands: wage earner, child care provider, elder care provider[4,14]

Racial and ethnic diversity of health care providers also plays a key role in providing care in underserved populations. In a cross-sectional analysis of more than 7000 adults by Marrast and colleagues[16] found that nonwhite physicians provided care to a disproportionate share of underserved populations. The growth of racially and ethnically diverse health care providers has not kept pace with the population growth in the United States. There is an opportunity to improve and address cardiovascular health needs that are often highest in underserved communities by increasing the number of racially and ethnically diverse providers in underserved communities.

Providers of all racial and ethnic backgrounds also need to be culturally competent for the populations in which they provide care. Cultural dynamics within a population should be assessed rather than assumed. Engaging community leaders, family members, and patients will provide information related to the health beliefs, values, and norms of the community.[16] These health beliefs will provide a foundation for the development of community-based interventions.

CLINICAL IMPLICATIONS

As previously noted, there is a high cardiovascular mortality among black men and a significantly higher prevalence of hypertension among the black population. Community-based interventions focused on hypertension management have demonstrated the most encouraging results in underserved populations.[12] This finding supports the idea that in the black population the focus in is still on treatment of chronic diseases such as hypertension, and that the emphasis needs to shift to improving cardiovascular health through risk reduction and behavioral change.

Recent analysis of the Joint National Committee 8 hypertension guidelines suggest that treating hypertension can result in the prevention of more than 50,000 cardiovascular events and 13,000 deaths.[13] This computer-simulated analysis was based on individuals aged from 35 through 74 years, and did not consider combined effects of concurrent implementation of other guidelines.[13] There are opportunities to enhance clinical outcomes through future analysis of population-based data that consider the possible synergistic effect of simultaneous use of multiple cardiovascular clinical guidelines.

Diverse community-based initiatives across the United States have sought to address many of these barriers, such as limited healthy food choices and safe places for increasing physical activity in creative ways. Reaching high-risk individuals requires innovation beyond imparting knowledge and recommendations for health promotion. Engagement in social marketing activities and community-based initiatives to improve access to nutritious food and safe places for activity are paramount to achieving success in these metrics.[4] Innovative strategies to enhance behavior change must be considered at the community level rather than relying on knowledge-based interventions. These initiatives should include using social media and phone technology to provide methods of communication that transcend physical boundaries.[4] The SMS Text-message Adherence support (StAR) trial is a 3-arm parallel, randomized clinical trial implementing a phone-based text-message system to focus on hypertension management in low-resource areas in South Africa.[17] This trial is focused on improvement in systolic blood pressure during a 12-month period while monitoring treatment adherence and additional quality measures. The significance of this trial is that patients are being recruited from primary care clinics in low- to middle-income settings, are typically seen in a "chronic disease lifestyle clinic," and are managed by nurse practitioners and physicians. This type of clinical environment mimics many of the clinics in medically underserved areas of the United States. Another key component of the StAR study is that hypertension treatment is congruent with both national and international guidelines.[17]

Additional strategies that have been deemed successful include community engagement at a grass-roots level. Barbershops, hair salons, and churches have been identified as places where community engagement can be successful in addressing the needs of individuals and families in an underserved population.[18] Both individual and group support may occur in any of these venues and may be sustainable based on prior relationships.

In a community-based randomized controlled study of 525 patients from a federally qualified health center focused on cardiovascular risk reduction, participants were assigned to 1 of 2 groups; usual care by primary provider or a nurse practitioner/community health worker (NP/CHW) team that focused on individualized behavioral, pharmacologic, and lifestyle interventions, with phone contact between clinic visits.[19] Clinical outcome measures mirrored those identified by the AHA focused on cardiovascular health, and included blood pressure, hemoglobin A_{1c}, and lipids.[7,19] The NP/CHW teams implemented the cardiovascular clinical guidelines for the management of diabetes, hypertension, and hyperlipidemia.[19] The results of this study indicated that for this medically complex underserved population the NP/CHW team effectively addressed cardiovascular risk factors in a comprehensive manner which was cost effective.[19] These findings support a team-based model of care inclusive of nursing and community health workers for underserved populations.

The use of electronic health records (EHR) provides an opportunity for patients to receive written information regarding strategies to improve their health at the conclusion of a clinical encounter. These EHRs prompt the provider to include health promotion education in addition to disease-specific information. The use of health-related applications for smartphones provides real-time resources for patients within the context of their daily activities. Providing diverse forms of patient education including Web sites, toll-free phone numbers, and smartphone applications allows this information to be used with patients of all ages and resources (**Table 3**).

Table 3
Patient resources for improving health behaviors and reducing cardiovascular risk

Topic	Examples of Patient Resources
Smoking	CDC - How to Quit Smoking - Quit Tips (www.cdc.gov) 1-800-QUIT-NOW Free phone-based information SmokefreeTXT (http://smokefree.gov/SmokefreeTXT/) Tips and advice for teens *Smoke free apps* (available in IOS and Android) QuitStart NCI QuitPal Quit Guide
Healthy diet and weight reduction	The American Heart Association's Diet and Lifestyle Recommendations (www.heart.org) DASH diet (www.dashdiet.org) 7-d Heart-Healthy Meal Plan (www.eatingwell.com) *Diet apps* (available in IOS and Android) Fooducate Calorie Counter and Diet Tracker by MyFitnessPal Eat Slower
Social support	*Social Support apps* Heart 360 Coach: provides information to improve heart health. Comprehensive tracking of blood pressure, cholesterol, glucose, weight, medications, and physical activity weLost: A social weight loss network Healtheo360: individuals with chronic conditions support one another

SUMMARY

Identification of cardiovascular risk should begin during early adolescence so that health promotion activities can be addressed and disease prevention strategies enacted. From an epidemiologic perspective vulnerable populations demonstrate the highest prevalence of cardiovascular disease, and should be the focus of prevention models.

The downstream effect of high cardiovascular mortality and morbidity affects quality of life, disability, and overall health of many underserved communities where the risk is highest. Patient empowerment is one of the key components of introducing any type of therapeutic lifestyle change related to cardiovascular risk reduction.[20] Community engagement is necessary to address the current barriers that exist, and using the AHA 7 metrics of cardiovascular health provides quantifiable factors to measure improvement. Using a multifaceted approach can yield incremental success in improving cardiovascular health in vulnerable populations.

REFERENCES

1. Brown TM, Parmar G, Durant RW, et al. Health professional shortage areas, insurance status and cardiovascular disease prevention in the reasons for geographic and racial differences in stroke (REGARDS) study. J Health Care Poor Underserved 2011;22:1179–89.

2. Arnett DK, Goodman RA, Halperin JL, et al. AHA/ACC/HHS strategies to enhance application of clinical practice guidelines in patients with cardiovascular disease and comorbid conditions, from the American Heart Association, American College of Cardiology and US Department of Health and Human Services. Circulation 2014;130:1662–7.

3. Stuart-Shor EM, Berra KA, Kamau MW, et al. Behavioral strategies for cardiovascular risk reduction in diverse and underserved racial/ethnic groups. Circulation 2012;125:171–84.

4. Bryant LL, Chin NP, Cottrell LA, et al. Perceptions of cardiovascular health in underserved communities. Prev Chronic Dis 2010;7(2):1–10.

5. Eckel RH, Jakicic JM, Ard JD, et al. 2013 AHA/ACC guideline on lifestyle management to reduce cardiovascular risk. A report of the American College of Cardiology/American Heart Association Task Force on practice guidelines. Circulation 2013;129:576–99.

6. Murphy MP, Coke L, Staffileno BA, et al. Improving cardiovascular health of underserved populations in the community with life's simple 7. J Am Assoc Nurse Pract 2015. http://dx.doi.org/10.1002/2327-6924.12231. 1–9.

7. Mozaffarian D, Benjamin EJ, Go AS. Heart disease and stroke statistics-2015 update. Circulation 2015;131:e29–322.

8. Ayanian JZ, Landon BE, Newhouse JP, et al. Racial and ethnic disparities among enrollees in Medicare advantage plans. N Engl J Med 2014;371:2288–97.

9. Melton KD, Foli KJ, Yehle KS, et al. Heart failure in Hispanic Americans: improving cultural awareness. J Nurse Pract 2015;11(2):207–13.

10. Go AS, Mozaffarian D, Roger VL, et al. Heart disease and stroke statistics—2014 update: a report from the American Heart Association. Circulation 2014;129(3): e28–292.

11. US Department of Health and Human Services, National Institutes of Health. SOL: Study of latinos. Hispanic community health study book. A report to the communities; Bethesda (MD): US Department of Health and Human Services, NIH, National Heart, Lung and Blood Institute; 2013. NIH Publication No. 13–7951.

12. Walton-Moss B, Samuel L, Nguyen T, et al. Community-based cardiovascular health interventions in vulnerable populations: a systematic review. J Cardiovasc Nurs 2014;29(4):293–307.

13. Moran AE, Odden MC, Thanataveerat A, et al. Cost-effectiveness of hypertension therapy according to 2014 guidelines. N Engl J Med 2015;372:447–55.

14. Laba T, Bleasel J, Brien J, et al. Strategies to improve adherence to medications for cardiovascular diseases in socioeconomically disadvantaged populations: a systematic review. Int J Cardiol 2013;167:2430–40.

15. Savage M, Dumas A, Stuart S. Fatalism and short-termism as cultural barriers to cardiac rehabilitation among underprivileged men. Sociol Health Illn 2013;35(8):1211–26.

16. Marrast LM, Zallman L, Woolhandler S, et al. Minority physicians' role in the care of underserved patients: diversifying the physician workforce may be key in addressing health disparities. JAMA Intern Med 2014;174(2):289–91.

17. Bobrow K, Brennan T, Springer D, et al. Efficacy of a text messaging (SMS) based intervention for adults with hypertension: protocol for the StAR (SMS Text-message Adherence suppoRt trial) randomized controlled trial. BMC Public Health 2014;14:28.

18. Victor RG, Ravenell JE, Freeman A, et al. Effectiveness of a barber-based intervention for improving hypertension control in black men: the BARBER-1 study: a cluster randomized trial. Arch Intern Med 2011;171(4):342–50.

19. Allen JK, Himmelfarb C, Szanton S, et al. Cost-effectiveness of nurse practitioner/community health worker care to reduce cardiovascular health disparities. J Cardiovasc Nurs 2014;29(4):308–14.

20. Scisney-Matlock M, Bosworth HB, Giger JN, et al. Strategies for implementing and sustaining therapeutic lifestyle changes as part of hypertension management in African Americans. Postgrad Med 2009;121(3):147–59.

Exploring Health Implications of Disparities Associated with Food Insecurity Among Low-Income Populations

CrossMark

Mary K. Canales, PhD, RN[a],*, Nancy Coffey, BA[b], Emily Moore, BA[c]

KEYWORDS

- Community-academic partnerships • Food insecurity • Low-income populations
- Qualitative research

KEY POINTS

- Food insecurity correlates with the development and exacerbation of chronic health conditions among low-income adults and children.
- Results from a qualitative focus group study with food-insecure parents of young children and agency staff working in the food assistance field reinforces how health and well-being are negatively impacted by food insecurity.
- Using social determinants of health framework, nurses can make positive strides to reduce health disparities associated with food insecurity among low-income populations.

INTRODUCTION

Research with priority populations has been emphasized and encouraged by the Agency for Healthcare Research and Quality (AHRQ), but research outcomes lag in their ability to identify evidence-based solutions to improve health care safety, quality, efficiency, and effectiveness.[1] AHRQ's priority populations, specified by the Congress in the Healthcare Research and Quality Act of 1999 (Public Law 106–129), include

The authors have no commercial or financial conflicts of interest related to this research project.

The authors acknowledge funding support from the University of Wisconsin-Eau Claire Office of Research and Sponsored Programs and the University of Wisconsin-Extension Eau Claire County.

[a] Department of Nursing, University of Wisconsin-Eau Claire, 105 Garfield Avenue, Eau Claire, WI 54702, USA; [b] University of Wisconsin Cooperative Extension, Eau Claire County, 227 1st Street West, Altoona, WI 54720, USA; [c] Feed My People Food Bank, 2610 Alpine Road, Eau Claire, WI 54703, USA

* Corresponding author.

E-mail address: canalemk@uwec.edu

women, children, racial and ethnic minorities, populations with special health care needs (those with chronic illness, disabilities, and end-of-life care needs), as well as the elderly, low-income, inner city, and rural populations.[1] This article focuses on 2 AHRQ-designated priority categories: the Hmong, an ethnic minority group, and low-income populations.

Target Population: Ethnic Minority

Hmong residents comprised the largest ethnic minority group in the county in which the study was conducted.[2] The Hmong served as a US ally in the Vietnam War from the 1960s to 1975.[3] The first Hmong migration of notable size to the United States began with the fall of Saigon and Laos to Communist forces in 1975.[4] Many from the Hmong group had worked with pro-American anti-Communist forces during the conflicts in Vietnam and Laos, and as a result, they were subject to violence and retribution. Many Hmong people escaped Laos to Thailand where they were incarcerated in refugee camps.[4] The Hmong group emigrated from Southeast Asia to the United States from 1975 to 1994, when the final refugee camps were closed.[4] It has been 40 years since the first Hmong refugees settled in western Wisconsin.[3] Despite immense progress in adapting to the culture and geographic differences, the journey to the United States and Wisconsin continues to be fraught with challenges.[3]

Economically, Hmong residents have made dramatic gains, because of a strong work ethic and dedication to education. However, more than one-third (36.2%) of Hmong county residents live at the federal poverty level.[5] Many older adults struggle with language barriers, which affect their employability. At present, for most Hmong youth, speaking basic English is not an issue[3]; however, significant differences in performance measures exist.[6] For example, recent local school district data indicate that Asian students lag behind white students in reading and math proficiency.[6] Specific county data on food insecurity among the Hmong population do not exist; however, poverty does increase the risk of food insecurity and hunger. As 36% of Hmong county residents are poor,[5] many of the poor are also likely to be food insecure. One unique issue for Hmong residents' food intake is that in their native countries, they ate fresh produce exclusively. This preference for fresh versus frozen or canned fruits and vegetables contributes an added cost to the food budget, especially in the winter (EC Hmong agency staff, personal communication, April 15, 2015).

Target Population: Low Income

According to the 2011 AHRQ national health disparities report, of all the measures of health care quality and access that are tracked and evaluated for trends over time, "poor individuals had worse care than high-income individuals in the most recent year for 52 measures" with most of these measures showing no significant change in disparities over time.[7(p244)] These health disparity trends persist today. According to the 2014 AHRQ quality and disparities report, few disparities have been eliminated and "people in poor households generally experienced less access to and poorer quality of care."[8(pvi)] To more accurately evaluate the impacts of food insecurity, the authors considered low income to be at 200% of poverty.[9] This is the percentage used by the federal government to set program eligibility thresholds for nutrition programs including Women, Infants, and Children (WIC) and Supplemental Nutrition Assistance Education (SNAP).[10] Based on this poverty threshold, 1 of 3, that is, 33%, of county residents where the study was conducted are considered to have low income.[11]

The US Department of Agriculture (USDA) definition of food insecurity,[12] a household-level economic and social condition of limited or uncertain access to adequate food, recognizes that access to healthy food is affected by social as well as economic conditions and therefore affects those above as well as below federal poverty thresholds. It is important for nurses to understand that many individuals and families who may not qualify for government-supported nutrition programs may still suffer from food insecurity.[13] In the authors' research, the USDA definition was used to ensure inclusion of the voices of parents with young children whose income may not meet federal definitions of low income but who may clearly live without access to adequate food.

Health Implications

With the health of low-income populations continuing to be disproportionately affected by disparities related to quality and access,[8] the authors' community-academic research team addressed one particular area, food insecurity. It is evident from multiple research studies that many health problems are associated with inadequate access to healthy food, from obesity and diabetes to cardiovascular disease and hypertension to depression,[14-16] with chronic health conditions exacerbated by food insecurity.

Eating nutritious foods is one of the major modifiable determinants of chronic diseases,[17] yet residents need supportive environmental and policy interventions to optimize access to affordable healthy food choices. Poverty puts households at a much higher risk of food insecurity.[18] Owing to the additional risk factors associated with poverty and food insecurity, low-income people are especially vulnerable to chronic diseases.[19,20] Recent research reported an association between adults in food-insecure households and a higher risk of hypertension and diabetes compared with those living in food-secure households[20] with other research linking food insecurity and increased risk for obesity.[19] These chronic health conditions further exacerbate low-income residents' ability to live healthy lives.

A recent study identified that nearly 1 in 3 US adults with a chronic disease has problems paying for food and/or medicine; chronically ill adults who reported food insecurity were much more likely to skip medication because of worries about cost than those who did not report problems affording food.[14] Another recent study reported that in a low-income population the risk for emergency department admission due to hypoglycemia increased 27% in the last week of the month compared with the first week.[20] The investigators suggested that exhaustion of food budgets might be an important driver of health inequities.[20] These and other results reinforce the importance for nurses to be cognizant of the relationships between the broader determinants of health, such as food insecurity and poverty, and their long-term impacts on chronic disease management.

In this article, a community-based research project is described whose aim was to qualitatively investigate perspectives of food insecurity from those directly affected by it: parents with young children residing in urban and rural areas of a midwestern state. The authors begin with an overview of the project team, describe the recruitment and data collection processes, discuss the results of the study, and conclude with recommendations for how nurses can collaborate, advocate, and intervene to address persistent disparities associated with food insecurity among low-income populations.

Setting

Located in Western Wisconsin, the county in which the study was conducted is home to 101,438 residents, including a city with 65,883 residents and small rural communities dispersed across 638 square miles.[2] The rural nature of the region and the large agricultural industry mask the reality that food insecurity exists. Food insecurity is often coupled with poverty, as in the study county, where the poverty rate is 14.7%, between the state average of 13.3% and the national average of 15.9%.[2] Among the Hmong population, the poverty rate is significantly higher, more than double the general county figure, at 36%.[5] In order to gain a better understanding of the impact food insecurity has on the health and well-being of families with young children, an academic-community research partnership was formed.

The partners included professionals from the regional food bank; a SNAP-Ed coordinator and Ameri-Corps VISTA from the county Extension office, including an employee who herself experienced food insecurity; and a nursing professor and students from the department of nursing at the local university. This interdisciplinary approach was essential for project success. To ensure that the voices of those who experience food insecurity as well as staff from local agencies who work to provide eligible families with food were heard, a community-based participatory approach was used.

RESEARCH PROCESS

Between fall 2011 and spring 2013, the research team met regularly, on an average 1 to 2 times per month, to develop and revise the consent forms, demographic questionnaire, and focus group questions; to plan, review, and revise recruitment processes; to host focus groups; and to analyze data.

Data Collection

Human subjects
Before data collection, every research team member completed human subject's certification training. The project itself was reviewed and approved by the sponsoring university's Institutional Review Board. Before the start of each focus group, the consent form and demographic questionnaire were completed by each participant. As part of the consent process, permission was obtained from each participant to digitally record the focus group discussion. As no participants objected, all focus groups were digitally recorded.

Data collection tools
The research team had multiple meetings to develop focus group questions and a demographic questionnaire. During question development and refinement, the research team gained valuable insights from the team member with personal food insecurity experience as well as state extension food insecurity specialists. State extension specialists also assisted in aligning demographic questions with existing food insecurity instruments.[21,22]

The initial set of focus group questions was organized according to key themes identified in an earlier community round table meeting, attended by residents, media representatives, and extension staff:

- Theme 1: Why are people hungry?
- Theme 2: What does it mean to be hungry?
- Theme 3: What is working? Suggestions?

Specific focus group questions were generated for each theme with probes to further explore the questions. Following a pilot group, the questions were revised based on feedback from the focus group facilitator, the team member who experienced food insecurity, and the focus group observer as well as on review of the transcript. This revised question set was used for all remaining focus groups with parents experiencing food insecurity. A separate set of questions was generated for the staff focus group, held after all parent focus groups were completed, to gain agency perspectives and parallels on the same themes.

Owing to the desire to compare the county WIC food insecurity survey data, obtained every 5 years, with the demographic questionnaire for parents experiencing food insecurity in this research project, the same USDA Household Food Security 6-question short form was used.[21] Questions were also asked about income, household numbers, and employment.[22] A separate, shorter demographic questionnaire was developed for staff participants.

Recruitment
Focus group methodology is valuable in gaining diverse perspectives on topics that often have been minimally examined[23] such as food insecurity among parents of young children. Although useful in collecting multiple views during a single encounter, there are many challenges in recruiting and ensuring participation in a focus group, especially concerning the sensitive topic of food insecurity. Although the authors anticipated that recruitment would be challenging and planned accordingly, they underestimated the vast difficulties that would be encountered.

Agency-specific recruitment approaches
Members of the research team were at the time of the study connected to many local community agencies and had relationships with staff working with families who experienced hunger. Building upon these relationships and working directly with community agencies proved to be the most successful recruitment approach. Parent participation in a focus group was much more likely when it included support and encouragement from someone they trusted.

Two groups held during summer 2012 used this approach and resulted in strong participation. One group (8 participants) was recruited from a local housing project and shelter, while the other group (10 participants) was recruited from the Family Literacy program and its partnering Head Start agency. Both groups were hosted at familiar, convenient locations with some transportation provided, which also increased participation rates.

Many factors contributed to the success of the Family Literacy-Head Start focus group. This group was composed of Hmong parents, who spoke little English, so that translation services were essential. The authors collaborated with the local Hmong assistance center; they provided space to hold the focus group and space for child care, and also paid translation services. The local Head Start provided an additional translator and a culturally appropriate lunch. The translators promoted the event, assisted participants to complete the demographic form, and translated the entire discussion. Although the research team's facilitator attended the group, her role was limited to providing assistance to those who spoke English. On-site child care eased parents' concerns; they knew their children were nearby. All of these facilitating factors were needed for focus group success.

School district recruitment approaches
The authors met as a research team during the summer to plan recruitment of parents from the local city school district and 1 rural school district. The city district was a large target group. A colorful bookmark with contact information was developed that was simple, inexpensive, and easily distributed. The authors purchased 7000 bookmarks and collaborated with the school district staff to distribute them to all district elementary school students through their backpacks during September 2012. Despite this vast outreach effort, the authors lacked direct connection to parents; subsequently, they received only 30 inquiries.

For the school district parent focus groups, the authors collaborated with the local children's museum. All the school district focus groups were held in the museum conference room, using the museum for child care. The authors collaborated with the local university's early childhood literacy program to provide childcare. Several different dates and times (day and evening) were offered to accommodate varying schedules. Participants were called or were sent e-mail reminders the day before the scheduled group. Despite all these efforts, only 19 participants attended.

Rural recruitment approaches

Hosting a rural focus group was also a challenge. Multiple recruitment efforts included a focus group notice in the school newsletter; bookmark distribution through children in kindergarten and first grade, the local food pantry, and library; and direct recruitment during the first class day at the elementary, middle, and high schools. The authors received only 10 inquiries with 4 participants attending the focus group.

In summary, the authors held 7 parent focus groups with a total of 43 parent participants over the course of 8 months (May to December 2012) and 1 focus group with 8 agency staff (**Table 1**). Despite extensive planning, varied recruitment strategies, and multiple participant incentives, more time, effort, and coordination were required than originally anticipated for recruiting parents who are food insecure. Although challenging data to collect, the results provide valuable insights for understanding the difficulties that food-insecure families experience.

Sample Description

Tables **2** and **3** summarize the demographic profile of the parent participants. The following were the key factors from respondents:

- Over half (56%) of the households interviewed had 2 children or less.
- Almost 68% had children aged 10 years or less (see **Table 2**).
- Most participants were couples or part of 3-generational households (see **Table 2**).
- Over half of the families had an annual income of $20,000 or less.

Table 1
Focus group data collection summary

Date	Focus Group Type	Number of Participants	Time	Location
May 7, 2012	Pilot group-parents	2	9–11 AM	Children's Museum
July 16, 2012	Hmong parent group	10	12–2 PM	Hmong Center
September 11, 2012	Housing Project & Abuse Shelter parent group	8	9–11 AM	Western Dairyland
October 3, 2012	City School district parent group	3	6–8 PM	Children's Museum
October 5, 2012	City School district parent group	9	12–2 PM	Children's Museum
October 19, 2012	City School district parent group	7	12–2 PM	Children's Museum
November 12, 2012	Rural School district parent group	4	9–11 AM	Rural Library-community room
March 15, 2013	Agency staff	8	3–4:30 PM	Hmong Center
Total	—	51 43 parents 8 staff	—	—

Table 2
Parent written survey data: household occupancy

Number of households with children <18 y	None	1–2	3–4	5 or More		No. of Participants
	1	23	13	6		43

Ages of children in household	0–2	3–5	10–12	11–13	14–17	No. of Participants
	10	24	31	19	12	96[a]

Number of adults per household	One	Two	Three			No. of participants
	12	28	3			43

Description of people in household	Single Mother/ Children	Single Father/ Children	Couple/ Children	Grandparents/ Children	3 Generations/ Children	Foster Parent/ Children	Others	No. of participants
	11	2	23	2	3	0	2	43

[a] Totals more or less than number of participants.

Table 3
Parent written survey data: coping with inadequate food

	Yes	No	If Yes				No. of Participants
			Almost every month	Some months, not every month	Only 1 or 2 mo	Unanswered	
Cut size or skipped meals because not enough food	36	7	18	15	3	7	43
Eat less than felt should because not enough food	34			No 9			43
Hungry because could not afford enough food	31	No 11		Unanswered 1			43

- About 42% reported cutting the size of meals or skipped meals almost every month because of insufficient food.
- About 40% could not afford balanced meals (see **Table 3**).

Most agency staff were women (8) who had worked in the field of food assistance from 1 to more than 15 years. Reasons for becoming involved in their work varied; for some it was "by accident," whereas for others, it was a life-long commitment toward improving the community for all residents (**Box 1**).

RESULTS
Analysis

Focus groups were digitally recorded and transcribed verbatim by members of the research team. The focus group with Hmong parents was more complex. Two Hmong interpreters, who were known and trusted by the participants, were hired to facilitate this focus group. One Hmong interpreter read the questions to the participants in Hmong, while the other interpreter interpreted participants' responses in English. Before transcription into English, the recording of this group was reviewed by the translator who had read the questions to confirm accuracy of the verbal English translation.

Because focus group questions were organized around themes originally identified in the earlier community round table, the initial coding also began with these themes. The research team met multiple times to discuss coding progress and refine the coding scheme. Individual team members coded a set of transcripts; these coding results were further reviewed and analyzed collectively. Using thematic analysis, the authors collapsed similar ideas into broader themes that reflected consistent patterns among the data.[23] Results are presented according to these broader themes.

Being food insecure affected all aspects of life. For the research participants, these effects revolved around the following 4 primary themes:

- Falling through the cracks
- Struggling physically and emotionally with hunger
- Juggling to meet life's basic needs
- Desiring healthy foods without the means

These 4 themes were consistent across the parent focus groups, including the Hmong participants. The Hmong participants shared experiences that were similar

---

Box 1
How staff participants became involved in their work

- Volunteered first
- Assumed full-time position w/school district
- Worked initially in private sector; hired into county supervisor position
- "It found me!" Started in field out of college, loved it, and has not left
- "Really by accident." Project management skills needed by nonprofit agency
- "Love for my community"
- "Love it!" Public health since college graduation
- Through work and colleague
- Began as preschool teacher and became interested in whole family; moved through different roles in effort to improve families' lives

to those expressed in other groups including frustration with government rules for assistance programs, increased stress, and the challenges of living in poverty. Hmong parent quotes are identified to highlight these similarities. It is also noteworthy that these themes were consistent among parent and staff participants. The quotes in **Table 4** highlight the consistency between the parent and agency staff participants across the 4 themes.

Of particular interest to nurses and the health care community in general is how medical issues and the subsequent need for treatment upended the often precarious balance families attempted to maintain. Issues related to medical conditions were evident across all 4 themes. **Table 5** outlines examples of how families and agency staff were impacted when health problems and food insecurity collided.

In conclusion, perceptions of parents experiencing food insecurity and the staff working with them were consistent. Both groups agreed that more needed to be done to address the gaps families experience in their efforts to access healthy, affordable food. The challenges are many, whereas the resources to improve the conditions in which many of these families live are often limited.

SUMMARY/DISCUSSION

Despite the impacts of food insecurity on all aspects of life, food insecurity is not readily visible to the community at large, including the health community. Four major themes were identified that reflected participants' experiences: falling through the cracks, struggling physically and emotionally with hunger, juggling to meet life's basic needs, and desiring healthy foods without the means. As these families attempted to manage their struggles, they also attempted to hide food insecurity from their own children. As one parent stated, *"Kids should be kids. They shouldn't feel our stress to worry about what we're gonna feed them or what they're gonna eat."* This face of hunger is critical for harnessing community commitment and engagement in tackling food insecurity issues.

Although critical, it is often difficult to hear directly from those experiencing hunger. While the authors learned from the participants about their experiences, they also learned some valuable lessons about reaching the target population and engaging them in the research process. These lessons may be applicable for nurses planning to conduct future research, develop community coalitions, or engage in other efforts that assist low-income residents experiencing food insecurity to improve their health.

Lessons Learned

Recruitment
The research team knew that recruitment would be a challenge, yet despite many community connections, incentives to compensate time and encourage participation, previous research experience, and some funding, recruitment proved to be more difficult than anticipated. Focus group methodology is not as simple as some may anticipate. The authors learned that successful recruitment methods include

- Hosting focus groups in a familiar place where staff in that location are trusted by participants.
- Linking focus group participation with an already existing program or group activity.
- Connecting directly with staff who work with the target population.

These recruitment methods were especially successful for connecting with the Hmong population. The Hmong focus group was held at the local Hmong agency serving the population. Participants were involved in an existing Head Start/Family Literacy program and were comfortable with the staff; translators who were known within the Hmong community were hired. Finally, a member of the authors' research team was well known to the staff from the Head Start/Family Literacy program and the Hmong agency, so strong connections were already in place. When combined, these recruitment methods led to the most successful group in terms of number of participants.

Several potential participants declined to participate when they understood it would be a group rather than an individual interview. Incorporating an individual interview option may be a useful strategy for reaching individuals willing to participate but reluctant to share in a group setting.

Stigma

Hunger and the experiences associated with food insecurity are very difficult topics to discuss even among others who share similar experiences. The stigma associated with being hungry and having difficulty feeding one's family was especially evident among rural parents, who were especially challenging to recruit into the study. Living in a small town, where it seems everyone knows everyone, increases the embarrassment for families who struggle to meet food needs. Engagement of rural participants could be facilitated through

- Direct connections between parents who experience food insecurity and trusted local rural agency staff, such as school counselors, school parent liaisons, and health department home visiting nurses
- Providing transportation to and from the focus group interview
- Offering the option of a one-on-one interview to rural residents instead of focus-group-only interviews, especially those experiencing transportation challenges

RECOMMENDATIONS

In order to eliminate persistent health inequities related to food insecurity, nurses and other health professionals need to direct efforts toward identifying food-insecure patients, increasing access to healthy food for low-income populations, and reducing the existing stigma associated with hunger. For these changes to occur, however, a community needs to be ready to hear the stories of those directly affected by food insecurity and motivated to engage in long-term strategic planning to realize change. According to Health in All Policies,[24(p1)]

> There is an increasing recognition that the environments in which people live, work, learn, and play have a tremendous impact on their health. Re-shaping people's economic, physical, social, and service environments can help ensure opportunities for health and support healthy behaviors. Solutions to our complex and urgent problems will require collaborative efforts across many sectors and all levels, including government agencies, businesses, and community-based organizations.

Nurses can play a key role in identifying "solutions to the complex and urgent problems" associated with food insecurity. The recommendations given in **Box 2** for addressing food insecurity are based on the focus group data, current evidence from the literature, and the authors' experiences working with low-income populations. Recommendations are ordered from least to most difficult to implement.

Nurses can be in the forefront to formalize, lead, and implement these health equity recommendations. With skills in collaboration, inherent trust among many

Table 4
Themes and corresponding data

Theme	Parent Participants	Agency Staff Participants
Falling through the cracks	There's no grace period...right now you're cut. That actually happened to me. This past spring I picked up contract work, 160 h was all they contracted me for and it was just enough to make me lose my food stamps. For the whole month of June, I lost all of them. So there's that hole that you fall into as soon as you report that income and it's never enough to make up the loss. (Parent) We cannot afford balanced meals because we fall into a gray area where we can't afford for the programs yet we don't have enough to be comfortable. It's not because, we're skinny, it's not because we choose to be. (Hmong parent)	I think there are a lot of families that are falling through the cracks, that don't qualify for programs, but still aren't able to feed their families, especially if they have children. They aren't necessarily homeless families or anything like that, but they're falling through the cracks
Struggling physically & emotionally with hunger	It's very different, because when there isn't enough, the stress level there is just super high, kids will be nagging, crying, and when you do have enough it is exactly the opposite, everybody is happy. (Parent) The stress level, when you don't have enough it makes, it's just unbearable, when even with an apple when you have to cut that up between all your kids with bag of ramen noodle when you have to divide everything up, it's just, and we live in the land of plentiful and we are starving. (Hmong parent)	I had a physician contact me who said, I can't, because of HIPPA, tell you who I'm sending, but we're sending an elderly person because, this was a Caucasian person, she did not want her children to know she didn't have enough money to buy groceries and she was eating cat food (others: ohhhh).

Juggling to meet life's basic needs	When we run short or food we go to food pantries, XXX (free meal site), just to…okay it's getting toward the end of the month. We're running short, we have to find ways to stretch it. But I don't have a car so getting around is another thing, so when I'm having to spend at the gas stations it goes quick so then you have to figure out how to stretch it the rest of the month. (Parent) It's very hard because, with transportation, because I could buy a used car that I can afford but it will break down in a month and it would end up being just as expensive as a new car to pay for but to get a new car I would not have the amount of money to pay for that and then you know after all the transportation expenses I would not have enough money just lying around for my kids. (Hmong parent)	But we're still seeing families in our neighborhood that if they chose to use their dollars for food or even for cleaning supplies, then they're faced with, at the end of the month, being short and not having enough money for housing; it's a constant juggle.
Desiring healthy foods without the means	What makes it hard for me is that I really want the kids to be able to eat healthy foods and, you know, plan out my meals and things like that but normally due to time constraints and things like that, I don't have the time to plan out the meals… I mean I would love to switch to organic vegetables, but financially that is completely out of the question and so that's a struggle for me every time I go shopping. (Parent) Sometimes I go lightheaded and I know it's because I don't eat balanced meals like they tell us when we go down to the places where we apply for these programs. (Hmong parent)	…getting to the food if you don't have a vehicle that works and you're relying on the city bus and you've got young kids. The best place downtown, for a lot of our families, is the little gas station where you're gonna spend a lot for your money for that kind of food and there's not a lot of healthy choices.

Table 5
Food insecurity and health

Theme	Participants' Perspectives
Falling through the cracks	...And we've been on and off of programs, and they've helped us, everything has always helped us. Currently, and our biggest thing right now is, as of September 1st we lost our medical assistance for myself and my husband. The children still remained on it because of the new sliding scale. Just when we think we are two steps ahead, we make too much money so now we're in this predicament where, do we pay $800 a month in his insurance through work which is more than I bring home a month, and then I'm working just, you know I love what I do... (Parent)
Struggling physically & emotionally with hunger	I have to go without some medications so that I can provide food for my kids too, you know. (Parent) I've run across a lot of people in that situation (going without medications), and that's hard because your kids need you to be healthy so that you're there for them, but then you have to give up medication in order to provide (another participant – to provide food for them, yep) food... (Parent) ...my blood sugars are up and down, up and down all throughout the day because I'm not getting the right nutrition, and that, I think, affects my daughter more than her own issues of I want this and not this, or I don't want spaghetti for the 4th day in a row [laughing], so my own mood is affected so greatly by it, that I think that is what's hardest for her is dealing with my mood swings. (Parent)
Juggling to meet life's basic needs	We both work and sometimes it is very misleading when people think that there is two incomes coming into the home that we're sustainable and that we are able to help ourselves more but there is the cost of having two of everything that has to work, gas, everything else that when you add it up we really have nothing at the end of the month. And let alone if somebody gets sick we have to go to the hospital and that is a mess by itself. And the copay it's expensive too and the premiums for Badger Care [Medicaid] as well. (Hmong parent) Badger Care costs are expensive and also if there's a complication at the clinic that Badger Care doesn't cover it so then it comes out of pocket. (Hmong parent) We've had people apply and one of the big obstacles for them are medical bills, and unfortunately, our applications don't take into consideration any medical bills. It's based on gross income, so that's tough for the families with medical issues. (Staff) I've heard that too where it doesn't take into consideration how much out of their pay goes to health insurance premiums (other staff: right) and how little they're actually getting in take home pay (other: right). (Staff)
Desiring healthy foods without the means	...you hear so many politicians complaining about childhood obesity and all of this, kind of, health issues and it all ties into health insurance and all of that stuff, but when you're on food stamps you need things that you can afford. Things like pasta that are going to fill you up too, but things that are going to make you gain weight...things that are going to fill you up, less healthy for you and you are going to probably gain weight and, in turn, have health problems, then the health insurance... (Parent) I think there's a big difference between eating and eating healthy. Now it's getting toward colds season and now my kids are gonna get sick because they don't get enough fruits or vegetables or vitamins or any kind because they're more expensive than candy bars [laughing]. (Parent)

Box 2
Recommendations for addressing food insecurity

Collaborate with local and regional media outlets to disseminate research outcomes and increase community awareness of and engagement with efforts to address food insecurity

Ensure voices of residents struggling with food insecurity are involved in community-wide hunger reduction plans including research, coalitions, and media events.

Examine how SNAP dollars are allocated and support pilot programs to optimize access and effectiveness of SNAP benefits for eligible families.[25,26]

Collaborate with local health entities including hospitals, insurance companies, and city-county health departments to strategically plan efforts to connect community residents' health to acquiring healthy affordable food.

Use a food security screening question in health care settings to enable staff to identify families in need of food resources and facilitate access to SNAP application and other available community assistance.[22]

Mobilize community stakeholders in an inclusive, nonprescriptive process requiring leading/learning-centered approaches to create and implement a strategic plan that aligns with the identified need.[27]

---

organizations and individuals, and the capacity to engage partners in coalition efforts, nurses are well positioned to become part of the solution to ending food insecurity and reducing persistent health disparities that disproportionately affect low-income populations.

REFERENCES

1. Priority populations. Agency for Healthcare Research Quality website. Available at: http://www.ahrq.gov/health-care-information/priority-populations/index.html. Accessed January 9, 2015.
2. State and County Quick Facts-Wisconsin. United States Census Bureau website. 2014. Available at: http://quickfacts.census.gov/qfd/states/55000.html. Accessed January 9, 2015.
3. Lindquist E. Old Hmong vs new Hmong. Eau Claire Leader-Telegram 2015;1A:9A.
4. Pfeifer ME. Hmong Americans. Asian-Nation: the landscape of Asian America website. 2003. Available at: http://www.asian nation.org/hmong.shtml. Accessed April 20, 2015.
5. Eau Claire County, Wisconsin, C17002 Ratio of Income to Poverty Level in the Past 12(Data). 2006–2010 American Community Survey Selected Population Tables for Hmong alone. U.S. Census Bureau website. Available at: http://factfinder.census.gov/bkmk/table/1.0/en/ACS/10_SF4/C17002/0500000US55035/popgroup~020. Accessed April 21, 2015.
6. Wisconsin Department of Public Instruction. Wisconsin Information System for Education Dashboard website. Available at: http://wisedash.dpi.wi.gov/Dashboard/portalHome.jsp. Accessed April 20, 2015.
7. Agency for Health Research Quality. National health disparities report 2011. Rockville (MD): Author; 2012. Available at: http://www.ahrq.gov/research/findings/nhqrdr/nhdr11/nhdr11.pdf.
8. Agency for Health Research Quality. National health quality and disparities report 2014. Rockville (MD): Author; 2015. Available at: http://www.ahrq.gov/research/findings/nhqrdr/nhqdr14/2014nhqdr.pdf.

9. U.S. low-incoming working families increasing. Population Reference Bureau website. 2015. Available at: http://www.prb.org/Publications/Articles/2013/us-working-poor-families.aspx. Accessed April 21, 2015.
10. Map the Meal Gap. Feeding America website. 2014. Available at: http://www.feedingamerica.org/hunger-in-america/our-research/map-the-meal-gap/2012/2012-mapthemealgap-exec-summary.pdf. Accessed April 21, 2015.
11. American fact finder: American Community Survey one year estimates. US Census Bureau website. Available at: http://factfinder.census.gov/faces/nav/jsf/pages/community_facts.xhtml. Accessed January 9, 2015.
12. Definitions of food security. USDA Economic Research Service website. 2010. Available at: http://www.ers.usda.gov/topics/food-nutrition-assistance/food-security-in-the-us/definitions-of-food-security.aspx. Accessed January 9, 2015.
13. Cook JT, Black M, Chilton M, et al. Are food insecurity's health impacts underestimated in the U.S. population? Marginal food security also predicts adverse health outcomes in young U.S. children and mothers. Adv Nutr 2013;4(1):51–61.
14. Berkowitz SA, Seligman HK, Choudhry NK. Treat or eat: food insecurity, cost-related medication underuse, and unmet needs. Am J Med 2014;127(4):303–10.e3.
15. Berkowitz SA, Karter AJ, Lyles CR, et al. Low socioeconomic status is associated with increased risk for hypoglycemia in diabetes patients, 2014: Study of Northern California (DISTANCE). J Health Care Poor Underserved 2014;25(2):478–90.
16. Kushel MB, Gupta R, Gee L, et al. Housing instability and food insecurity as barriers to health care among low-income Americans. J Gen Intern Med 2006;21(1):71–7.
17. Story M, Kaphingst K, Robinson-O'Brien R, et al. Creating healthy food and eating environments: policy and environmental approaches. Annu Rev Public Health 2008;29:253–72.
18. Curtis K, Bartfeld J, Lessem S. Poverty and food insecurity in Wisconsin and Eau Claire County. Madison (WI): Applied Population Laboratory; Department of Community & Environmental Sociology; University of Wisconsin-Madison; 2014. Available at: http://www.apl.wisc.edu/resource_profiles/pfs_profiles/eauclaire_2014.pdf.
19. Why low-income and food insecure people are vulnerable to overweight and obesity. Food Research and Action Center (FRAC) website. 2010. Available at: http://frac.org/initiatives/hunger-and-obesity/why-are-low-income-and-food-insecure-people-vulnerable-to-obesity. Accessed January 9, 2015.
20. Seligman HK, Laraia BA, Kushel MB. Food insecurity is associated with chronic disease among low-income NHANES participants. J Nutr 2010;140:304–10.
21. WIC Program, WIC, Nutrition & Physical Activity Section, Bureau of Community Health Promotion, Division of Public Health, Wisconsin Department of Health Services. Food insecurity in the Wisconsin WIC Population. Madison (WI): 2012. Available at: https://www.dhs.wisconsin.gov/wic/foodsecurity.pdf. Accessed January 9, 2015.
22. USDA-Economic Research Service. Six item short form for food security survey module. Washington, DC: 2012. Available at: http://www.ers.usda.gov/datafiles/Food_Security_in_the_United_States/Food_Security_Survey_Modules/short2012.pdf. Accessed January 9, 2015.
23. Polit DE, Beck CT. Nursing research: generating and assessing evidence for nursing practice. 9th edition. Philadelphia: Wolters Kluwer/Lippincott Williams & Wilkins; 2012.
24. Rudolph L, Caplan J, Ben-Moshe K, et al. Health in all policies: a guide for state and local governments. Washington, DC; Oakland (CA): American Public Health Association and Public Health Institute; 2013.

25. Jilcott SB, Wall-Bassett ED, Burke SC, et al. Associations between food insecurity, supplemental nutrition assistance program (SNAP) benefits, and body mass index among adult females. J Am Diet Assoc 2011;111(11):1741–5.
26. Wilde PE. Measuring the effect of food stamps on food insecurity and hunger: research and policy considerations. J Nutr 2007;137(2):307–10.
27. Fitzgerald N, Spaccarotella K. Barriers to a healthy lifestyle: from individuals to public policy—An ecological perspective. JOE 2009;47(1). Article 1FEA3. Available at: http://www.joe.org/joe/2009february/a3.php.

Assessing Health Issues in States with Large Minority Populations

 CrossMark

Michelle Long, MPH[a], Charles E. Menifield, MPA, PhD[b],
Audwin B. Fletcher, PhD, APRN, FNP-BC[c],*

KEYWORDS

- Health outcomes • Infant mortality • Obesity • Low birth weight
- Teenage pregnancy • Per capita health care spending • Minority population

KEY POINTS

- Regions with large minority populations have the highest average low birth, obesity, infant mortality, and teenage pregnancy.
- Regions with large minority populations have the lowest per capita health care spending rates.
- Statistical analysis reveals there are several variables policymakers can control via the policy-making process that could impact health outcomes.

INTRODUCTION

The term budget crisis has been at the forefront of many current events and political and economic discussions for some time. Health expenditures is often brought up as a contributing factor to this crisis, as the United States has witnessed significantly large increases in health care spending in recent decades. In 2010, per capita health expenditures were $8,402, more than 48% higher than that of the next highest spending country, Switzerland.[1] As such, it is easy to conclude that higher levels of spending would yield positive health outcomes. However, by most measures of health status, this is not the case.

Disclosure Statement: This article is not currently under review at another journal. If accepted, the authors fully intend for the article to be published by the journal *Nursing Clinics of North America*.
[a] Master of Public Health Program, University of Missouri, 804 Lewis Hall, Columbia, MO 65211, USA; [b] Truman School of Public Affairs, University of Missouri, 121 Middlebush, Columbia, MO 65203, USA; [c] University of Mississippi Medical School of Nursing, 2500 North State Street, Jackson, MS 39216, USA
* Corresponding author.
E-mail address: afletcher@umc.edu

Recent research indicated teenage pregnancy and infant mortality rates have decreased by several percentage points over the last 2 decades.[2–4] These decreases raised the main question for this research: are governmental efforts to curtail negative health outcomes and social problems working? Hence, a study was proposed to assess the relationship between per capita state health care expenditures and several health outcomes (infant mortality, obesity, low birth weight, and teenage pregnancy). More specifically, the authors were interested in comparing per capita health care spending in states with large minority populations to changes in the aforementioned outcomes in 5-year increments beginning in 1990; this led to the following research question: Is there a relationship between per capita health care spending and location of a state as it relates to various health outcomes? This question is an important one because the evidence indicated southern states tend to have poorer health outcomes. In the bigger scheme of health care finance, the authors also wanted answers to some more general questions, such as: Should health care spending be more targeted toward specific outcomes? Are there special characteristics about states that cause the outcomes to vary? Are there policy decisions that can promote a healthier state?

LITERATURE REVIEW

Although there is much research examining health outcomes,[5,6] the authors focused their attention on research that examined health outcomes and spending at various levels of analysis (individual, country, and so on). Using data from the Organization for Economic Co-Operation and Development (OECD), Anderson and Poullier[7] found per capita health care spending in the United States ($3925) far surpassed that of any other of 18 nations (developed) in the data set. The next closest country was Switzerland at $2547. Anderson and Poullier[7] also found that health care spending as a percentage of gross domestic product (GDP) was highest in the United States at 13.5% in 1997 compared with a low of 4% in Korea and Turkey. Compared with the United States, the researchers found infant mortality was higher and life expectancy was lower in Korea and Turkey.[7] Bokhari and colleagues[8] found in a more recent country level analysis that health care expenditures do improve health outcomes with substantial variations across countries. For example, allocating funds for more hospital staff could improve health outcomes, but these efforts may be thwarted if the quality and quantity of roads in the country do not coincide with those changes.

Anderson and colleagues[9] also discussed spending patterns and poor health outcomes and suggested high rates of chronic illness in the United States could be a contributing factor to rising costs. Although insightful and relevant, neither Anderson and colleagues[9] nor Anderson and Poullier made claims about causation or use statistical analysis to support their claims.[7]

Hadley and colleagues[10] found a relationship between health care spending and better health outcomes, suggesting cuts in health care among poorer elderly could result in poorer health.[10] Although a quasi-experimental study, this study differed from most of the other studies the authors examined in their study. In fact, the study was one of the few found with a statistically significant correlation between spending and outcomes. Perhaps this is due to the specific population (elderly) Hadley and colleagues examined.

In contrast to Hadley's findings, Gupta and colleagues[11] found (using a cross-sectional study with data from 70 countries) low-income persons generally have worse health outcomes than higher income individuals. The researchers also concluded that health spending alone will not significantly improve the health status of the poor, but it remains an important variable. When considering specific variables, for example, they found that a 1% increase in health expenditures reduced infant mortality by twice as many deaths among the poor. They also found that primary school enrollment and economic growth models that included private resources for health care were positive contributors to health outcomes.

Using OECD cross-national data, Filmer and colleagues[12] assessed the impact of nonhealth factors and public spending on infant and child mortality. First, the researchers found 95% of the variation in under-five mortality was explained by income, income distribution, female education, and other cultural factors. Second, Filmer and colleagues[12] found income as a solitary independent variable was a significant factor, but other factors were equally important in explaining this outcome. Last, the researchers found higher levels of public health care spending, as a share of GDP, was "tenuously related to improved health status."[12(pp39)] Overall, they found that the impact of public spending on health was small.

More often than not, the most common thread in the research is the lack of causality.[13] That is, does the absence of increased spending result in poorer health outcomes? Although some literature does exist regarding the relationship between health care spending and health outcomes as it pertains to societal well-being, there is still need for a more comprehensive look at multiple variables affecting health outcomes. Hence, this current analysis expands on the current literature by including social, demographic, and economic variables in one model to explain effects of per capita health care spending. (See also Centers for Disease Control and Prevention [CDC]. [2009]. Case studies: low birthweight. Pediatric and pregnancy nutrition surveillance system. Available at: http://www.cdc.gov/pednss/how_to/interpret_data/case_studies/low_birthweight/what.htm. Centers for Disease Control and Prevention. [2012]. Overweight and Obesity. Available at: http://www.cdc.gov/obesity/. Centers for Disease Control and Prevention. [2013]. Reproductive Health. Available at: http://www.cdc.gov/reproductivehealth/index.htm. United Health Foundation. [2012]. America's Health Rankings. Available at: http://www.americashealthrankings.org/. The Organization for Economic Cooperation and Development. Assessment of Health Care in Four Countries. Available at http://www.oecd.org/home/0,2987,en_2649_201185_1_1_1_1_1,00html, Accessed March 3, 2011.)

DATA AND METHODS

The objective of this study was to determine the relationship between per capita state health care spending on health outcomes. Thus, the authors collected state-level data from a variety of sources for all 50 states for the period 1990 to 2010 (N = 950) (**Box 1**, bullet 1). Data sources for obesity, teenage pregnancy, infant

---

Box 1
Data and method additional facts

- Although the authors used data from 1990 to 2010, data were not available for the entire period for every variable. Therefore, the number of cases for each model may vary.

- The phrase per capita health care spending refers to the average amount of dollars spent on each person in a state for any given year.

- Research shows that policy changes in 1 year are not reflected in the data for that year. In some cases, the law may change late in the year. Therefore, as many scholars have done, the authors lagged the dependent variable. For example, changes in policy that affect infant mortality that were passed into law in 2009 were not likely to be seen until 2010. Hence, the authors use 2010 infant mortality data with 2009 independent variables.

mortality, low-birth-weight (LBW) rates, and their other independent variable were retrieved from the Centers for Medicare and Medicaid Services, the US Bureau of Economic Statistics, the United Health Foundation, Centers for Disease Control and Prevention, Department of Education, Statistical Abstract of the United States, The National Center for Health Care Statistics, and the US Census Bureau. The authors used SPSS,(version 21, and Excel to conduct their statistical analysis).

The authors began their analysis by first examining the trend pattern (graph) of each of the dependent variables with the independent variable, state-level per capita health care spending (see **Box 1**, bullet 2), in 5-year increments. The authors then tabulated the average obesity, infant mortality, teenage pregnancy, and LBW by regions and compared each with the national average. The key independent variable studied was per capita health care expenditures. The dependent variables were time-lagged infant mortalities, obesity rates, teen pregnancy rates, and LBW rates (see **Box 1**, bullet 3).

Because state level panel data were used in the analysis, the authors used fixed effects regression models to examine how a series of independent variables affected each of the dependent variables. Thus, the authors included dummy variables for state, year, and the total population to account for differences across states and time that the might not be explained by the other variables in the model. To control for extraneous variables, the authors used a variety of relevant control variables. However, all of the variables were not included in each model. In addition, the authors used previous research as well as intuition to guide the selection of the variables. For example, it seemed rational that urban transit ridership may affect obesity levels, whereas it may not explain teenage pregnancy rates.

The control variables included the following: race (% of the white population); graduation rates (high school graduation); poverty rates; region (South and non-South); income (per capita income); uninsured (% of uninsured population); SPH (% of single-parent households); Medicaid (% of the population enrolled in Medicaid); smoking (% of the population over the age of 18 that smoke); PCHS (per capita state health care spending); hospitals (number of hospitals); doctors (number of doctors); fruits and vegetables consumption; APC (adequacy of prenatal care); BSM (births to single mothers); physical activity (% of the population who engage in physical activity); and urban transit ridership (% of persons using urban transit); sex education (courses in public schools); and HIV education.

The regression models were expressed as follows:

Lagged Obesity Rates = Per Capita Health Care Spending + Region + White Population + Income + Poverty + Medicaid + Smoking + Graduation + Hospitals + Uninsured + Fruits and Vegetables + Urban Transit + Physical Activity + Error.

Lagged Teenage Pregnancy Rates = Per Capita Health Care Spending + Region + White Population + Income + Poverty + Medicaid + Smoking + Graduation + Hospitals + Adequacy of Prenatal Care + Uninsured + Sex Education + HIV Education + Single Parent Household + Error.

Lagged Infant Mortality Rates = Per Capita Health Care Spending + Region + White Population + Income + Poverty + Medicaid + Smoking + Graduation + Hospitals + Uninsured + Fruits and Vegetables + Low Birth Weight + Teenage Pregnancy + Adequacy of Prenatal Care + Physical Activity + Single Parent Household + Error.

Lagged   Low   Birth   Weight   Rates   =   Per   Capita   Health   Care
Spending + Region + White Population + Income + Poverty + Medicaid +
Smoking   +   Graduation   +   Hospitals   +   Uninsured   +   Fruits   and
Vegetables + Teenage Pregnancy + Adequacy of Prenatal Care + Single Parent
Household + Physical Activity + Doctors + Hospitals + Births to Single
Mother + Error.

FINDINGS

For each of their 4 dependent variables, the authors first provide a graph depicting the
dependent variable and per capita health care spending. This analysis is followed with
a table showing the dependent variable with regional averages by year. Last, the authors provide a regression model showing the relationship between their dependent
variable with their per capita health care and region variables as well as numerous
control variables.

INFANT MORTALITY

Fig. 1 depicts the infant mortality from 1990 to 2010 and the corresponding per capita
health care spending variable in the United States. The data indicate infant mortalities
have declined consistently over the period. In 1990, the average infant mortality in the
United States was roughly 9.1%, and 6.2% in 2010. Conversely, per capita health care
spending in the United States increased incrementally over the same time period. In
fact, per capita health care spending was roughly $2570 per person in 1990 and
$7000 per person in 2010.

    Table 1 shows the average infant mortalities every 5 years for the period 1990 to
2010 for each of the regions. Although the US and regional averages dropped

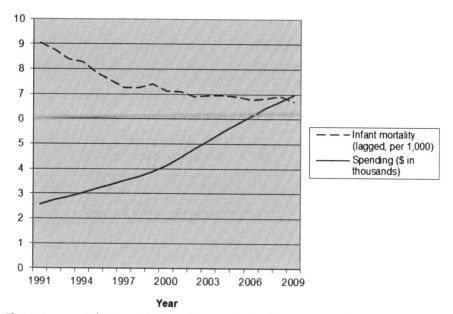

Fig. 1. Average infant mortalities and per capita health care expenditures in the United
States.

Table 1
Average infant mortalities by year and region

Region	1990	1995	2000	2005	2010
South	10.63	9.15	8.66	8.35	7.54
Southwest	8.58	6.48	6.38	6.2	5.83
Midwest	9.11	7.84	7.23	6.87	6.43
West	8.45	6.84	6.46	6.18	5.45
Northeast	8.51	7.06	6.55	6.12	5.84
National average	9.06	7.55	7.09	6.75	6.22
Minimum	6.2 (ME)	5.2 (MA)	4.6 (MA)	4.7 (VT)	3.75 (AK)
Maximum	12.4 (GA)	10.5 (MS)	10.7 (MS)	9.6 (MS)	9.7 (MS)

precipitously during each period, the disparity between the southern region and the rest of the country was quite noticeable. In fact, the southern region was over a full percentage point higher than any other region during each period. Mississippi, the highest ranked state in the latter 4 periods, was more than 3 percentage points higher than the US average and nearly 6 percentage points higher than the lowest ranked state of Alaska in 2010.

When the authors considered their main independent variables in the infant mortality regression model (**Table 2**), which contains numerous control variables, they found a more complete picture of the impact of per capita health care spending. As highlighted in italics, the authors noted that as per capita health spending increased, infant mortalities increased. The variable was significant at the 0.000 level. This level of significance indicated the level of predictability in their model was at the highest level and hence they have correctly identified a variable that affected their dependent variable.

Table 2
Infant mortality regression model

	Coefficient	Std. Error		Coefficient	Std. Error
White population	−0.013^c	(0.003)	*Region (South vs Non-South)*	*0.254^a*	*(0.125)*
Per capita income	−2.932E−5^c	(0.000)	Fruits and vegetables	−0.005^a	(0.003)
Poverty rates	−0.014	(0.014)	LBW	0.409^c	(0.043)
Medicaid enrollment	2.774E−9	(0.000)	Teenage pregnancy rate	0.034^c	(0.006)
Smoking (over 18)	0.062^c	(0.014)	Adequacy of prenatal care	0.017^b	(0.006)
Per Capita State Health Care Spending	*0.000^c*	*(0.000)*	Physical activity	0.004^a	(0.003)
HS Graduate Rate	0.017	(0.015)	Single parent household	0.008	(0.013)
Hospitals (no.)	0.001	(0.001)	Total uninsured population	−0.045^c	(0.001)
Constant	88.596^a	(46.038)	Adj. R^2	0.628	—
F	58.365^c	N		647	—

Note: The model includes a year, state, and total population variable for the fixed effects.
  [a] Significant at the 0.05 level.
  [b] Significant at the 0.01 level.
  [c] Significant at the 0.00 level.

In addition, the authors found their regional variable was also significant because southern states were more likely to have a higher infant mortality. The authors also found infant mortalities decreased as the white population, fruit and vegetable consumption, per capita income, and total uninsured rates increased. Conversely, the data also revealed that as smoking, physical activity, teenage pregnancy, adequacy of prenatal care, LBW, and per capita health care spending increased, infant mortality increased. Last, the F coefficient (58.365) was significant as well as the adjusted R^2 (0.628).

OBESITY

The data in **Fig. 2** depict obesity rates for each year from 1990 to 2010 along with per capita health care expenditures in the United States. In addition, the data indicated obesity rates increased each year during this period. More specifically, the obesity rate increased from 11.7% in 1990 to 27.7% in 2010 in the United States. In comparison to changes in the US obesity rate, the slope of the line for per capita health care spending in **Fig. 2** shows a slower growth pattern. Again, the average per person health care spending average in 1990 was $2570 and $6970 in 2010.

Table 3 displays the average obesity rates every 5 years from 1990 to 2010 for each region. The table shows a consistent increase in the rate for each region and each period. The southern region had the highest rate for each period and grew at a faster rate than the remaining regions. This data reveal the south was different than the remaining regions as the gap has widened over time. Again, Mississippi led all states with an average rate that was roughly 7 percentage points higher than the national average.

Table 4 provides the regression model for obesity. It is notable in the data findings that obesity rates increased as per capita health care spending increased. Again, the authors noted that the region variable is significant as it indicated southern states had higher rates of obesity. The analysis also revealed obesity rates decreased as the

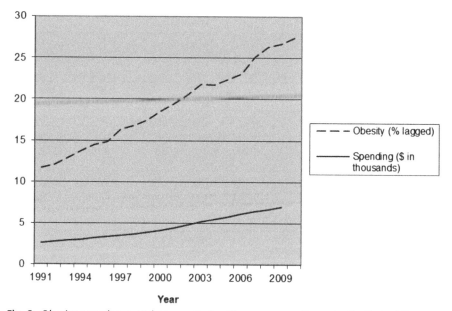

Fig. 2. Obesity prevalence and per capita health care expenditures in the United States.

Table 3
Average obesity rates by year and region

Region	1990	1995	2000	2005	2010
South	12.77	16.79	22.01	26.07	31.18
Southwest	11.35	13.45	19.13	22.3	26.28
Midwest	11.69	15.93	19.68	23.44	28.72
West	10.88	14.18	18.63	21.91	25.75
Northeast	11.57	13.62	18.16	21.83	26.45
National average	11.65	14.88	19.46	23.09	27.71
Minimum	6.9 (CO)	6.2 (DE)	13.8 (CO)	16.7 (CO)	21.4 (CO)
Maximum	15 (MS)	19.6 (IN)	24.4 (MS)	29.4 (MS)	34.5 (MS)

white population, urban transit ridership, fruit and vegetable consumption, total uninsured population, and high school graduation increase obesity rates increased. In addition, the data show obesity rates increased as per capita income, smoking, and the number of hospitals increased. The adjusted R^2 was 0.813, indicating that the model explains 81% of the variance using these variables. Last, the F coefficient was very high at 177.352, indicating a strong relationship between the variables.

TEENAGE PREGNANCY

Fig. 3 depicts teenage pregnancy rates from 1990 to 2010 along with per capita health care spending. During this 20-year period, teenage pregnancy rates decreased consistently through 2004 and leveled off. Concurrently, per capita health care spending has more than doubled during the period.

Table 5 shows the average teenage pregnancy rate by region and year for the period 1990 to 2010 in 5-year increments. The data indicate that the rate decreased each year during the period. In fact, the US average decreased by 22.8 pregnancies

Table 4
Obesity regression models

	Coefficient	Std. Error		Coefficient	Std. Error
White population	−0.018[b]	(.007)	Region (South vs Non-South)	.746[c]	(.264)
Per capita income	0.000[c]	(0.000)	Fruits and vegetables	−0.029[c]	(0.006)
Poverty rates	0.006	(0.032)	Physical activity	0.007	(0.006)
Medicaid enrollment	−1.053E−007	(0.000)	Total uninsured population	−0.103[c]	(0.026)
Smoking (over 18)	0.213[c]	(0.029)	HS graduate rate	−0.161[c]	(0.032)
Hospitals (no.)	0.015[c]	(0.002)	Urban transit ridership	−0.014[c]	(0.003)
Per Capita State Health Care Spending	0.000[a]	(0.000)		—	—
Constant	−2211.090[c]	(100.138)	*Adj. R^2*	0.813	—
F	177.352[c]	*N*		649	—

Note: The model includes a year, state, and total population variable for the fixed effects.
  [a] Significant at the 0.05 level.
  [b] Significant at the 0.01 level.
  [c] Significant at the 0.00 level.

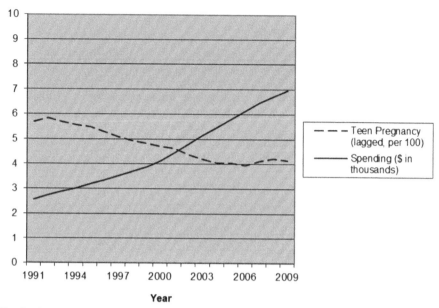

Fig. 3. Average teenage pregnancy rates and per capita health care expenditures in the United States.

since 1990. Although the southwest region in the United States maintained the highest average teen pregnancy rate, Mississippi remained at or near the top of the charts during each year of the analysis. The northeast region had the lowest average rate. Overall, the range between the rates dropped steadily for the 5 regions over this 20-year period.

The regression model in **Table 6** shows teenage pregnancy rates decreased as the white population, Medicaid enrollment, per capita state health care spending, high school graduation rates, and adequacy of prenatal car increased. The region variable was also significant, indicating that the southern region had higher rates of teenage pregnancy. Last, teenage pregnancy rates increased as smoking, the total uninsured population, single parent household, hospitals, and sex education courses in schools increased. The F value (171.182) and the adjusted R^2 (0.785) coefficients woro vcry high, indicating a strong relationship between the variables.

Table 5
Average teen pregnancy rates by year and region

Region	1990	1995	20,000	2005	2010
South	72.97	68.67	61.96	51.70	44.24
Southwest	75.58	74.90	66.68	57.88	46.53
Midwest	54.36	50.16	44.23	34.45	33.82
West	52.76	46.38	39.98	35.61	32.23
Northeast	44.21	41.48	35.12	28.56	24.09
National average	56.8	52.7	46.2	39.4	34.0
Minimum	33 (NH)	28.6 (VT)	23.4 (NH)	17.9 (NH)	15.7 (NH)
Maximum	81.0 (MS)	80.6 (MS)	72.0 (MS)	61.6 (NM)	55.0 (MS)

Table 6
Teenage pregnancy regression models

	Coefficient	Std. Error		Coefficient	Std. Error
White population[a]	−0.109[c]	(0.023)	Region (South vs Non-South)	2.571[c]	(0.816)
Per capita income	−2.770E−005	(0.000)	Single parent household	0.479[c]	(0.086)
Poverty rates	0.077	(0.099)	Adequacy of prenatal care	−0.208[c]	(0.041)
Medicaid enrollment	−1.297E−006[b]	(0.000)	Hospitals (no.)	0.050[c]	(0.006)
Smoking (over 18)	0.250[b]	(0.083)	Sex education	2.304[b]	(0.671)
Per capita state health care spending	−0.003[c]	(0.000)	HIV education	0.400	(0.564)
HS graduate rate	−0.733[c]	(0.088)	Total uninsured population	1.073[c]	(0.089)
Constant	−112.778[c]	(9.436)	Adj. R²	0.785	—
F	171.182[c]		N	747	—

Note: The model includes a year, state, and total population variable for the fixed effects.
[a] Significant at the 0.05 level.
[b] Significant at the 0.01 level.
[c] Significant at the 0.00 level.

LOW BIRTH WEIGHT

The data in **Fig. 4** indicate the LBW trend from 1990 to 2010. As shown, the LBW rate increased at a slower rate than health care spending. In fact, the data indicate LBW rate increased gradually over the period and slightly decreased in recent years. This

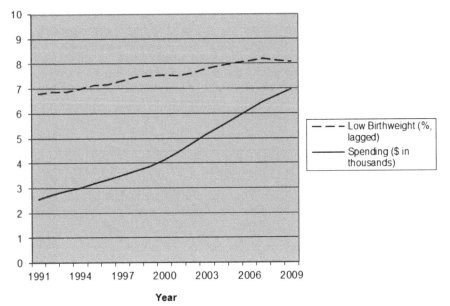

Fig. 4. Low birthweight prevalence and per capita health care expenditures in the United States.

Table 7
Average low birth weight rates by year and region

Region	1990	1995	2000	2005	2010
South	8.35	8.75	9.18	9.91	9.73
Southwest	6.98	7.2	7.4	8.0	8.13
Midwest	6.66	7.09	7.46	8.15	7.84
West	5.74	6.0	6.48	6.84	7.03
Northeast	6.57	7.1	7.29	7.88	7.89
National average	6.78	7.17	7.52	8.10	8.10
Minimum	4.8 (AK)	5.3 (AK)	5.6 (AK)	6.1 (AK)	5.7 (AK)
Maximum	9.6 (MS)	9.8 (MS)	10.7 (MS)	11.8 (MS)	12.1 (MS)

recent decrease was consistent with increased per capita health care spending over the same period.

Table 7 shows average LBW rates in the United States by year and region. The data indicate LBW increased consistently in every region over the period. The southern region during this period consistently maintained the highest LBW average rates throughout this 20-year period. For example, in 2010, the average LBW rate in the south was 1.63% higher than the national average. This finding was consistent across each period. The west region consistently had the lowest average LBW rate. When the authors examined each state, they noted that Mississippi led the country in LBW during each of the periods. Last, the gap between Mississippi and the US average has grown in recent years.

The LBW regression model in **Table 8** shows LBW increased as per capita health care spending increased. In addition, the southern region variable was significant in

Table 8
Low birth weight regression models

	Coefficient	Std. Error		Coefficient	Std. Error
White population	-0.008^a	(0.004)	Region (South v. Non South)	1.159^c	(0.129)
Per capita income	$4.716E-005^c$	(0.000)	Fruits and vegetables	-0.013^c	(0.003)
Poverty rates	-0.020	(0.015)	Births to single mothers	0.009	(0.005)
Medicaid enrollment	$-6.014E-008$	(0.000)	Teenage pregnancy rate	0.031^c	(0.007)
Smoking (over 18)	0.032^a	(0.016)	Adequacy of prenatal care	-0.004	(0.006)
Per capita state health care spending	0.000^a	(0.000)	Physical activity	0.004	(0.005)
HS graduate rate	-0.041^a	(0.017)	Single parent household	0.073^c	(0.015)
Hospitals (no.)	0.001	(0.001)	Doctors in state	0.004^c	(0.001)
Total uninsured population	-0.041^b	(0.015)	—	—	
Constant	-109.205	(60.304)	Adj. R^2	0.665	—
F	45.363^c	N		447	—

Note: The model includes a year, state and total population variable for the fixed effects.
[a] Significant at the 0.05 level.
[b] Significant at the 0.01 level.
[c] Significant at the 0.00 level.

Region	1991	1995	2000	2005	2009
South	$2483	$3121	$3994	$5376	$6420
Southwest	$2375	$2807	$3484	$4986	$5936
Midwest	$2577	$3188	$4121	$5791	$6814
West	$2416	$2961	$3902	$5582	$6817
Northeast	$2823	$3561	$4622	$6624	$7986
National average	$2567.30	$3186.70	$4122.62	$5810.00	$6970.42
Minimum	$1993.21 (UT)	$2341.56 (UT)	$3030.19 (UT)	$4346 (UT)	$5031 (UT)
Maximum	$3324.2 (CT)	$4134.21 (MA)	$5148.59 (MA)	$7436 (MA)	$9278 (MA)

Table 9
Average per capita health care spending rates by year and region

the expected direction. The data also indicate LBW decreased as the white population, high school graduation rates, total uninsured population, and fruit and vegetable consumption increased. Furthermore, LBW rates increased as per capita income, smoking, teenage pregnancy, single parent households, and doctors in a state increased. The adjusted R^2 was 0.665, explaining 66% of the variance in the model.

STATE HEALTH CARE SPENDING

Table 9 provides the data for average state health care spending by year and region from 1991 to 2009. The data reveal health care spending increased consistently over the period. In fact, average US spending nearly tripled during the period for each of the regions. Utah had the lowest average, whereas Massachusetts had the highest per capita spending.

SUMMARY

The main objective of this study was to determine the impact of per capita state health care spending on various health outcomes as well as to determine if region was important in understanding differences in health outcomes. More specifically, the authors wanted to determine if there were variations in health outcomes when the authors examined regions of the country that had large minority populations.

When the authors examined each of their dependent variables separately, they noted teenage pregnancy rates and infant mortalities decreased steadily over the 20-year period as per capita health care spending increased. However, LBW babies and obesity rates increased exponentially as per capita health care spending increased over time. In fact, per capita health care spending nearly tripled over the 20-year period of the study. What was notable from this analysis was the southern region had the highest LBW rates, highest infant mortalities, highest obesity rates, and the second highest teenage pregnancy rates (southwestern region was the highest) when compared with the other regions in the United States. On the surface, this descriptive analysis suggests regions with higher African American and Hispanic populations warrant more attention from policymakers and bureaucrats. More specifically, the descriptive data for states like Mississippi suggest obesity are nearing an epidemic level.

When the authors examined the data in the regression models, they found health care spending was related to health outcomes, but often in the wrong direction. That is, the regression models show obesity, LBW, and infant mortalities increased as per capita state health care spending increased. However, these findings were not completely surprising because it was expected that spending would be higher in areas where the rates were higher. This finding was also consistent with previous research by Anderson and Poullier,[7] who argued that health care spending did not necessarily yield desirable results in many cases.[7] However, the authors do note that growth in per capita health care spending was not consistent over the 20-year period. The south and southwestern regions consistently received less funding, but by 2010, this disparity increased and likely could explain some of the variance in the regression analysis.

Overall, their regression models consistently provide evidence for other factors that should be considered when constructing models to improve health outcomes in a state or region. These factors include the white population; the percentage of smokers over 18; region; fruit and vegetable consumption; the number of doctors in a state; the number of hospitals in a state; and, so on. The fact that the authors found multiple significant variables in their models made the case for a comprehensive approach to reducing health outcomes. Specifically, they first noted per capita health care spending was very high in regions and states that often had above average health outcomes. Although the cost of living in these areas was likely higher, bureaucrats and policymakers should revisit the funding structures for health care spending. The fact that Utah had the lowest per capita health care spending ratio and less than average health outcomes, in a positive sense, provided evidence that the current funding structure was not functioning at an optimal level. That is, other factors have to be analyzed in order to best create a scenario that is likely to yield the best results.

Although the authors make a good case to examine these health outcomes in a comprehensive manner, the data also suggested the outcomes should be examined independently of the remaining variables. For example, the urban ridership variable in the obesity model clearly showed that obesity levels decreased when people used public transportation. This finding seemed logical because people often have to walk to a specific location in order to use public transportation. Hence, for states with high obesity levels, this seemed to be one way to change the direction of that variable. In addition, the data showed fruit and vegetable consumption had a positive impact on lowering obesity rates. Again, this finding suggests that policymakers should strongly consider increasing healthier options in public schools and examine the number and location of grocery stores in metropolitan areas because the data suggest that food deserts tend to exist in poor communities.

The authors' analysis was not without limitations. Predominant among the limitations was the level of the data. Ideally, analysis of this type was better suited for individual, neighborhood, city, or county level data because regions within a state or city can change drastically when race, income levels, education rates, and so forth are considered. In addition, future research should consider additional variables such as economic development in the regions as well as political affiliations of elected officials.

REFERENCES

1. Key information on health care costs and their impact. Health care costs: a primer. Henry J. Kaiser Foundation. Available at: http://kff.org/health-costs/issue-brief/health-care-costs-a-primer/. Accessed May 12, 2012.
2. Menifield CE, Dawson J. Infant mortality in southern states: a bureaucratic nightmare. J Health Hum Serv Adm 2008;31(3):385–402.
3. Stampfel C, Kroelinger CD, Dudgeon M, et al. Developing a standard approach to examine infant mortality: findings from the state infant mortality collaborative (SIMC). Matern Child Health J 2012;16:S360–9.

4. Bell ER, Glover L, Alexander T. An exploration of pregnant teenagers' views of the future and their decisions to continue or terminate their pregnancy: implications for nursing care. J Clin Nurs 2014;23(17/18):2514–26.
5. Long EF, Brandeau ML, Owens DK. Potential population health outcomes and expenditures of HIV vaccinations strategies in the United States. Vaccine 2009; 27(39):5402–10.
6. Farag M, Nandakumar AK, Wallack S, et al. Health expenditures, health outcomes and the role of good governance. Int J Health Care Finance Econ 2013; 13(1):33–52.
7. Anderson G, Poullier J. Health spending, access, and outcomes: trends in industrialized countries. Health Aff 1999;18(3):178–92.
8. Bokhari FA, Gai Y, Gottret P. Government health expenditures and health outcomes. Health Econ 2007;16:257–73.
9. Anderson G, Frogner B, Reinhardt U. Health spending in OECD countries in 2004: an update. Health Aff 2007;26(5):1481–9.
10. Hadley J, Waidmann T, Zuckerman S, et al. Medical spending and the health of the elderly. Health Serv Res 2011;46(5):1333–61.
11. Gupta S, Verhoeven M, Tiongson ER. Public spending on health care and the poor. Health Econ 2003;12(8):685–6.
12. Filmer D, Hammer J, Pritchett L. Child mortality and public spending on health: how much does money matter? Policy research working papers. Washington, DC: World Bank; 1997. http://dx.doi.org/10.1596/1813-9450-1864.
13. Gupta S, Verhoeven M, Tiongson E. The effectiveness of government spending on education and health care in developing and transition economies. Eur J Polit Econ 2002;18(4):717–37.

APPENDIX

Definitions

This article uses the following health terms that will be described here. Globally, *infant mortality* is a commonly used, standardized indicator of a society's general health. The CDC defines infant mortality rate as "an estimate of the number of infant deaths for every 1000 live births" (2012).

Obesity is a standardized label for a range of body weight that is considered unhealthy for a given height (CDC, 2012).

The measurement for *smoking* used in this article is the percentage of the population over age 18 that smokes cigarettes regularly. According to the United Health Foundation, "regularly" is defined as self-reporting having smoked at least 100 cigarettes in a lifetime and currently smoking every day or some days. (Behavioral Risk Factor Surveillance System; 2012).

The term *teen pregnancy* is used to mean the number of births to women between the ages of 15 and 19 for every 1000 women in this age range (CDC).

Low birth weight is described by the CDC as a baby being born weighing less than 2500 g (5 lbs. 8 oz.) (2009).

Fruits and Vegetables is the percentage of the population that consumed fruit 2 or more times per day and vegetable 3 or more times per day (Behavioral Risk Factor Surveillance System).

Physical Activity is the percentage of the population that engaged in physical activity as recommended by the state (Behavioral Risk Factor Surveillance System).

Urban Transit Ridership is per capita urban transit ridership (National Transit Database).

Sex Education in Public Schools and *HIV Education in Public Schools* were taken from National Association of State Boards of Education and is the response to the question: Is sex education mandated in the public schools? (https://www.guttmacher.org/statecenter/spibs/spib_SE.pdf).

Region Dummy: South = Alabama, Arkansas, Florida, Georgia, Kentucky, Louisiana, Mississippi, North Carolina, South Carolina, West Virginia, Virginia, and Tennessee; Non-South = Arizona, New Mexico, Oklahoma, Texas, Missouri, Kansas, North Dakota, South Dakota, Illinois, Indiana, Iowa, Nebraska, Ohio, Michigan, Wisconsin, Minnesota, Colorado, Hawaii, Alaska, California, Oregon, Utah, Idaho, Montana, Wyoming, Nevada, Washington, Maine, Vermont, New Hampshire, Rhode Island, Maryland, Connecticut, Maryland, New York, Delaware, New Jersey, Massachusetts, and Pennsylvania.

Best Practices for Effective Clinical Partnerships with Indigenous Populations of North America (American Indian, Alaska Native, First Nations, Métis, and Inuit)

CrossMark

Emily A. Haozous, PhD, RN[a],*, Charles Neher, BS[b]

KEYWORDS

- American Indian • Alaska Native • First Nations • Métis • Inuit
- Culturally-congruent • Best practice • Disparities

KEY POINTS

- Health care delivery in indigenous communities must be culturally tailored to that specific community.
- Trust and communication are critical for successful clinical relationships with patients from American Indian/Alaska Native, First Nations, Métis, and Inuit communities.
- In regions where distance or rural location is a barrier to care, identify opportunities to use patient navigators, community health representatives/workers, and take advantage of resources such as telehealth to expand access to speciality care.
- Culturally congruent care emerges from collaborative relationships that recognize, respect, and honor indigenous values and worldviews.

INTRODUCTION

This article provides a review of the literature to identify best practices for effective clinical partnerships with indigenous populations of North America. Through collaboration, experience, and trial and error, clinicians and researchers have provided suggestions on best practices for collaborations with indigenous populations based on

Conflict of Interest: The authors have no conflicts of interest to disclose.
[a] College of Nursing, University of New Mexico, MSC 07 4380 Box 9, 1 University of New Mexico, Albuquerque, NM 87131-0001, USA; [b] MSC 07 4380 Box 9, 1 University of New Mexico, Albuquerque, NM 87131-0001, USA
* Corresponding author.
E-mail address: ehaozous@salud.unm.edu

lessons learned. This information will contribute to improving clinical practice in American Indian, Alaska Native (AI/AN) communities in the United States and First Nations, Métis, and Inuit communities in Canada to improve health outcomes and decrease health disparities.

BACKGROUND

In North America there are 2.9 million people identified as AI/AN alone in the United States and more than 1.5 million indigenous people in Canada, including First Nations, Métis, and Inuit.[1–3] There is wide diversity within these populations, and each AI/AN and indigenous Canadian community has its own unique cultural identity. This article will present information with the caveat that the interested clinician or researcher is best prepared by taking the time to learn the cultural and health-related specifics to the community in which they are working. Likewise, in the United States, federally recognized tribes are sovereign nations, and exist in a government-to-government relationship with the US federal government. Sovereign nations operate as independent entities within the boundaries of other governmental bodies, and mandate that the terms of original treaties that were negotiated as part of the delineation of tribal lands be honored as law.[4] Sovereign nations also dictate the administration of any policies regarding their land, resources, culture and citizens, commonly referred to as self-determination.[5]

Indigenous Canadian populations lack the formal government-to-government status of AI/ANs. Instead, some communities have formal self-governance agreements with the Canadian government, with full governmental bodies responsible for all tribal matters. Other communities are in a development phase as they grow into more mature government systems.[6] Although all indigenous Canadians do not have the same political and legal standing with the Canadian government, they do share the desire for self-determination.[7]

The indigenous peoples of the United States and Canada include the very rural reservation-dwelling populations as well as the most urban populations residing in large clusters in most major cities in the United States and Canada.[3–8] Although the health care needs of the indigenous patient change based on the populations' proximity to resources, many of the cultural needs remain static, and the barriers to caring for an urban population in Seattle are remarkably similar to those caring for a community in rural Montana.

OVERVIEW OF HEALTH STATISTICS

Although a border separates the 2 nations, health disparities are common across the indigenous populations of North America. Canadian indigenous populations experience heart disease at a rate 1.5 times higher than the general Canadian population; incidence of type 2 diabetes is 3 to 5 times higher, and the rates of tuberculosis infection are 8 to 10 times higher than in the Canadian general population.[9] AI/ANs are slightly more likely to die from heart disease and cancer than all races in the United States, but deaths from diabetes mellitus are 1.5 times higher, and rates of mortality from chronic liver disease and cirrhosis are 2.8 times higher than those of all races in the United States.[10]

METHODS

The authors reviewed the literature that focused on the lessons learned in collaborating with indigenous populations in the context of research and the clinical setting.

Articles were limited to those available in English with full text available, and characterized the elements necessary for effective research and clinical partnerships with indigenous populations. See **Box 1** for a complete list of search terms used. The authors reviewed all articles and extracted information related to lessons learned and implications for research and clinical practice. To compile best practices, the authors examined the literature and organized the information into the 2 large themes: conceptual guidelines and health care delivery (**Fig. 1**).

Conceptual Guidelines

There is a large body of literature showing that mortality and morbidity rates in AI/AN and Canadian indigenous populations are worse than rates for non-Hispanic whites. These disparities emerge from inequities within the clinical setting, including inadequacies in the relationship between providers and patients. Evidence-based practice suggests the importance of effective partnerships between clinical providers and indigenous communities/patients as a means of overcoming these disparities by improving patient engagement, provider investment in their patients, and better clinical recommendations. In reviewing the literature, 4 major conceptual themes were identified that characterize best practices for effective partnerships between clinical providers and indigenous communities/patients. The literature review also provided several suggestions for best practices in which to deliver health care to indigenous communities:

- Establish trusting relationships with those communities
- Work with each community as a unique tribal body, to include honoring the governmental structure of that community
- Consider culturally congruent communication in its many forms
- Collaborate with the community honoring indigenous values for successful outcomes

Clinicians and researchers emphasize the importance of a trusting, respectful relationship with staff and community as the primary cornerstones to successful

---

Box 1
Search terms used

- Lessons learned
- Indians, North American
- Alaska Native
- First Nations
- Aboriginal Canadian
- Clinical collaborations
- Research collaborations
- Academic tribal collaborations
- Cultural competency
- Clinical care
- Community-based participatory research
- Tribal sovereignty
- Self-determination

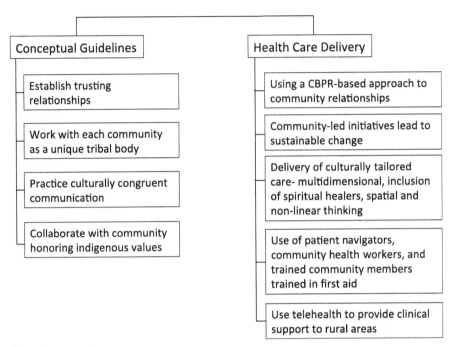

Fig. 1. Best practices.

outcomes. Trust is meaningful for both sides of the partnership, and authors have many suggestions for relationship building. Historically, indigenous communities have been exploited in research or had health policies imposed upon them without consultation, creating an atmosphere of mistrust. In order to address this historic legacy, trust building requires time and patience from both the community and the outside partner.[11,12] Trust is also easier to establish if the outside partner is able to spend physical time with members of the community in order to become known in the community, and to learn the local politics, culture, and issues important to people in the community.[11,13–16] Having a presence in the community also allows people a chance to know who the clinician or researcher is as a person, which can contribute to increased trust from the community.[17,18]

Another component of relationship building is the consideration of tribal leadership in clinical and research matters. Indigenous communities operate as autonomous entities and require the inclusion of relevant tribal leadership with any important clinical matters. When a new project is to be instituted at a community clinic, or a research program is proposed, the chief, tribal chair, tribal council, tribal health council, and other appropriate leadership should be consulted and kept informed throughout the process.[11,13,19] Transparency in communication allows the tribal leadership the opportunity to better understand the health priorities faced by the members of the tribe, which can in turn drive policies and resource allocation. Transparency also builds trust between the tribal members and the clinical staff and/or researchers.[16]

Communication is a foundation for positive clinical and research outcomes. Along with communication with tribal leadership, communication with the community through regular presence, responsiveness to community requests, and learning to communicate within the cultural norms of that tribe are all the responsibility of clinicians and researchers.[14,20–22] When working in or with an indigenous population, trusted clinicians can become part of the fabric of the community, and may be invited to ceremonial or community events. Malone[23] describes the phenomenon of boundary crossings, in which the clinician has established a trusting relationship, and remains aware of his or her role in the community to avoid crossing professional boundaries by going Native and inadvertently committing ethical violations. The outside clinician or researcher must remain professional and aware of his or her primary role in the community, whether that is to collect data or deliver health care.[23,24]

Communication is the cornerstone of most clinical encounters, yet communication in indigenous communities can vary from the mainstream. Oral traditions and storytelling are both valued, and have clear implications for clinical practice.[23] For example, communication of important health information is often expected to take place through spoken exchanges. In western health care, documentation takes place via written consent forms, but for many tribal people, signing documents indicating consent is disrespectful or is a challenge to the person's integrity.[25,26] There may be protocols for who can speak to whom, and clinicians should keep this in mind, especially in communities in which medical assistants are used to collect private health information. There may be cultural rules regarding the appropriateness of a young person asking sensitive questions of an elder.[26]

AI/AN and Canadian indigenous communication is frequently characterized by its storytelling elements. Communication through storytelling is a key feature in oral traditions, and permeates all aspects of many indigenous cultures in North America. Researchers have found that respecting storytelling and the integrity of the whole story aids in building a deeper understanding of the phenomenon of interest as well as deepening relationships with communities.[17,20,27] Clinicians observe that storytelling in the clinical encounter can include extensive information unrelated to what the nonindigenous clinician would consider relevant to the clinical problem.[22] Understanding the importance of the role of storytelling to the cultural context is critical in building trust, increasing overall communication, and may have important implications to patient engagement and clinical practice.

Cultural values vary widely across indigenous groups, but many share an interconnected, community-focused ontology that fundamentally sets them apart from the western culture.[17,22,23] Although this cultural value exists on a spectrum, the presence of this value is vitally important for clinical care, as it affects how health care decisions are made within a community. The individual patient may be experiencing the health problem, but care decisions may place the health of the community as the priority before that of the individual.[28,29] Likewise, any health care policies that are presented to tribal leadership will be considered at the community level.[23]

Health Care Delivery

Successful health care delivery in AI/AN and Canadian indigenous communities has several common features. Culturally congruent health care has several commonalities:

- Using a community-based participatory research (CBPR)-based approach to collaborative relationships
- Understanding that sustainable change comes from community-led initiatives
- Striving to deliver care that is tailored to meet the cultural needs of the specific community
- Use of patient navigators or community health workers
- Training rural community members in first aid
- Using telehealth resources for consultation and training of clinicians in rural areas

With the understanding that for many, community is the core unit of the indigenous identity, the practice of CBPR has contributed a new approach to collaborative research and clinical relationships with indigenous populations. As CBPR has been adopted as the best practice for ethical research in indigenous communities, AI/AN and Canadian indigenous communities alike have come to expect all collaborative relationships to mirror the key qualities of CBPR. This includes community–clinic partnerships via tribal health boards, valuing traditional wisdom through the use of spiritual leaders and incorporating traditional medicine as a healing modality,[7] and culturally tailoring clinic materials and teaching styles to meet the community's needs and priorities (**Box 2**).[15,23]

In a CBPR study designed to reduce childhood obesity conducted with tribes in North Carolina, authors found that the best means of ensuring sustainability was strong partnerships with tribal leadership.[13] In this project, partnerships included frequent written updates and presentations with tribal councils, engagement with tribal leaders for feedback throughout the program implementation, and responding to that feedback by tailoring the program to each community as appropriate. The research team also took care to stay connected with the tribes as leadership changed throughout the duration of the project, and educating the tribal leaders of the health concepts critical to the success of the project.

Although partnerships are critically important, the most sustainable health changes are often observed to come from within the community itself. As Begay[30] and Barnard[22] observed, it can be the role of the clinician to facilitate a change process that is already underway within a community in response to an observed clinical problem. For a clinician entering an indigenous community from the outside, the impulse may be to institute changes based on clinical practices standard in the general population. Several authors experienced in working with indigenous communities caution against this approach, with the reminder that every tribe is unique; interventions have to meet the cultural needs of the community, and there is existing knowledge within the community that must be recognized.[22,23,31]

Begay[30] presented a case study in which there was a strong need for a community-wide response to domestic violence in a small community on the Navajo reservation. Through mobilization of key stakeholders in the region, a coalition of volunteers formed that included community members, clinicians, and social workers. This

---

Box 2
Key principles of community-based participatory research

1. Recognizes community as a unit of identity

2. Builds on strengths and resources within the community

3. Facilitates collaborative partnerships in all phases of the research

4. Integrates knowledge and action for mutual benefit of all partners

5. Promotes a colearning and empowering process that attends to social inequalities

6. Involves a cyclical and iterative process

7. Addresses health from both positive and ecological perspectives

8. Disseminates findings and knowledge gained to all partners

From Israel BA, Schulz AJ, Parker EA, et al. Review of community-based research: assessing partnership approaches to improve public health. Annu Rev Public Health 1998;19:173–202; with permission.

volunteer coalition was able to build a dialogue within the community about domestic violence through health fairs, community meetings, and participation in community events. They were ultimately able to open a women's shelter, creating the infrastructure for safety for women living with violence in the process.[30]

Health care delivery in indigenous communities can have a distinctively different look and feel than mainstream health care. Culturally tailored health care takes into consideration region, values, and the priorities of the unique community being served. Many indigenous communities have been observed to conceptualize health as having distinctive yet complimentary domains, commonly categorized into physical, mental, emotional, and spiritual domains.[22,28,32,33] Clinicians delivering culturally tailored care are mindful of these domains and are inclusive of spiritual and emotional care as part of the clinical visit. Many tribal clinics will also include traditional healers on staff in order to address the spiritual healing components of their patient population.[7,24]

Clinicians working in indigenous communities are also observant of cultural differences in the perception of time. Where the western approach to clinical practice is to establish appointment times and expect dialogue to progress in a linear fashion, many indigenous individuals and communities have a broader and more extended sense of time and spatial sense. This has clinical implications for the clinician who expects a clinical day to run on a rigid schedule, or to have a clinical encounter to include a linear recounting of a patient's personal health history. Although this generalization is not to be applied to all indigenous populations, the clinician or researcher hoping to practice culturally congruent care is best advised to investigate where his or her community of interest falls on the spectrum of time and place orientation (**Box 3**).[22,29,32]

One approach that has been found to useful in managing cultural issues in communication between clinician and indigenous communities is through the use of patient navigators. Patient navigators are trained to guide patients through the health care system, and are especially useful for helping maneuver patients through unfamiliar health care systems. Navigators are particularly useful for patients in need of specialty care, such as patients diagnosed with cancer.[34] Patient navigators often come from the community, so they are able to act as intermediaries between the jargon-rich world of specialty care and that of the patient's home community. Many communities also employ community health workers, who act as a local resource to help transport patients to health appointments, provide basic health information, and who can be trained to do simple health checks such as blood glucose and blood pressure monitoring.[35]

The rural nature of many indigenous communities has presented a critical issue for those communities regarding access to basic and specialized health care. In addition to using community health workers and patient navigators, another strategy is to train community members in basic first aid. In places where access to a health care is

---

Box 3
Key features of culturally tailored care

- Unique to each community
- Considers how the community conceptualizes health
- Includes spiritual and emotional care as part of each clinical visit
- Consultation with traditional healers as appropriate
- Understand that community members may have different orientations to time that will impact the manner in which they interact with the clinical setting

prohibitive due to geography, providing training in first aid in order to fill a critical health care gap has proven extremely successful.[18] Vanderburgh and colleagues provided 2 intensive 5-day courses in first aid to individuals from a remote First Nations community in sub-Arctic Canada with a full-time nursing station but no on-site physicians or paramedics and the closest hospital 4 hours away by airplane. The success of this program relied on the ability of the trainers to adapt the program to the cultural and pedagogical needs of the community.[18]

Another approach to reaching remote rural indigenous communities is through the use of telehealth. Using videoconferencing, expert specialists are able to consult in real time with clinicians on site in rural areas, bridging a gap in care for patients who are unable to travel to an urban area to consult with specialty care. Haozous and colleagues demonstrated that clinicians attending telehealth grand rounds on cancer-related pain had significantly higher levels of user satisfaction and clinician confidence compared with those clinicians who did not attend the telehealth grand rounds.[36] The benefit of telehealth is that clinicians can access the sessions without having to leave their clinical practice to travel to a professional meeting, substantially decreasing time and economic burden on the clinics and communities.[37]

SUMMARY

Through this review of the literature, several best practices for collaboration in AI/AN and indigenous Canadian communities have emerged:

- Establish trusting relationships
- Work with each community as a unique tribal body
- Practice culturally congruent communication
- Collaborate with community, honoring indigenous values
- Use a CBPR-based approach to community relationships
- Support community-led initiatives for sustainable change
- Identify qualities that could contribute to the delivery of culturally tailored care
- Identify opportunities to use patient navigators, community health representatives or workers, and take advantage of human capitol when distance or other resources limit access to health care
- Use telehealth to connect clinicians working in remote areas to specialty care experts

Although many barriers still exist that contribute to persistent health disparities in AI/AN and Canadian indigenous communities, clinical innovations, ethical research, and relationship building with clinicians, academic centers, and researchers may contribute to improved indigenous health in the future.

ACKNOWLEDGMENTS

Funding for this manuscript was provided by the Robert Wood Johnson Foundation Nurse Faculty Scholars program grant #69347.

REFERENCES

1. Securing our futures. National Congress of American Indians. Available at: http://www.ncai.org/Securing_Our_Futures_Final.pdf. Accessed January 10, 2015.
2. Aboriginal peoples in Canada: First Nations people, Métis, and Inuit: National Household Survey. Statistics Canada. 2011. Available at: http://www12.statcan.gc.ca/nhs-enm/2011/as-sa/99-011-x/99-011-x2011001-eng.pdf. Accessed January 5, 2015.

3. Norris T, Vines PL, Hoeffel EM. The American Indian and Alaska Native population: 2010. 2010 Census Briefs. 2010; # C2010BR-10.

4. Steinman E. Settler colonial power and the American Indian sovereignty movement: forms of domination, strategies of transformation. Am J Sociol 2012; 117(4):1073–130.

5. Cook S. What is Indian self-determination? Red Ink Magazine 1996;3(1). Available at: http://faculty.smu.edu/twalker/samrcook.htm. Accessed January 5, 2015.

6. Governance. Aboriginal Affairs and Northern Development Canada. 2013. Available at: https://www.aadnc-aandc.gc.ca/eng/1100100013803/1100100013807. Accessed January 3, 2015.

7. Mundel E, Chapman GE. A decolonizing approach to health promotion in Canada: the case of the urban aboriginal community kitchen garden project. Health Promot Int 2010;25(2):166–73.

8. Aboriginal Affairs and Northern Development Canada. Fact sheet—urban aboriginal population in Canada. 2010. Available at: http://www.aadnc-aandc.gc.ca/eng/1100100014298/1100100014302. Accessed December 28, 2015.

9. Health Canada: First Nations and Inuit health. Health Canada. 2014. Available at: http://www.hc-sc.gc.ca/fniah-spnia/diseases-maladies/index-eng.php. Accessed January 12, 2015.

10. Espey DK, Jim MA, Cobb N, et al. Leading causes of death and all-cause mortality in American Indians and Alaska Natives. Am J Public Health 2014; 104(S3):S303–11.

11. Adams A, Miller-Korth N, Brown D. Learning to work together: developing academic and community research partnerships. Wis Med J 2004;103(2):15–9.

12. Lopez ED, Sharma DK, Mekiana D, et al. Forging a new legacy of trust in research with Alaska Native college students using CBPR. Int J Circumpolar Health 2012;71(18475):1–7.

13. Fleischhacker S, Byrd RR, Ramachandran G, et al. Tools for healthy tribes: improving access to healthy foods in Indian Country. Am J Prev Med 2012; 43(3S2):S123–9.

14. Ritchie SD, Wabano MJ, Beardy J, et al. Community-based participatory research with Indigenous communities: the proximity paradox. Health Place 2013;24: 183–9.

15. Tilburt JC, James KM, Koller K, et al. Assessing follow-up care after prostate-specific antigen elevation in American Indian/Alaska Native men: a partnership approach. Prog Community Health Partnersh 2013;7(2):153–61.

16. Kaufman CE, Black K, Keane EM, et al. Planning for a group—randomized trial with American Indian youth. J Adolesc Health 2014;54:S59–63.

17. Lavallée LF. Practical application of an indigenous research framework and two qualitative indigenous research methods: sharing circles and Anishnaabe symbol-based reflection. Int J Qual Methods 2009;8(1):21–40.

18. VanderBurgh D, Jamieson R, Beardy J, et al. Community-based first aid: a program report on the intersection of community-based participatory research and first aid education in a remote Canadian Aboriginal community. Rural Remote Health 2014;14(2537):1–8.

19. Kelley A, Belcourt-Dittloff A, Belcourt C, et al. Research ethics and indigenous communities. Am J Public Health 2013;103(12):2146–52.

20. Simonds VW, Christopher S. Adapting western research methods to indigenous ways of knowing. Am J Public Health 2013;103(12):2185–92.

21. Kimes CM, Golden SL, Maynor RF, et al. Lessons learned in community research through the Native Proverbs 31 health project. Prev Chronic Dis 2014;11:130256.

22. Barnard AG. Providing psychiatric-mental health care for Native Americans: lessons learned by a non-Native American PMHNP. J Psychosoc Nurs Ment Health Serv 2007;45(5):30–5.
23. Malone JL. Ethical professional practice: exploring the issues for health services to rural Aboriginal communities. Rural Remote Health 1891;2012(12):1–10.
24. Scurfield RM. Healing the warrior: admission of two American Indian war-veteran cohort groups to a specialized inpatient PTSD unit. Am Indian Alsk Native Ment Health Res 1995;6(3):1–22.
25. Baydala LT, Worrell S, Fletcher F, et al. "Making a place of respect": lessons learned in carrying out consent protocol with First Nations elders. Prog Community Health Partnersh 2013;7(2):135–43.
26. Naqshbandi M, Harris SB, Macaulay AC, et al. Lessons learned in using community-based participatory research to build a national diabetes collaborative in Canada. Prog Community Health Partnersh 2011;5(4):405–15.
27. Christensen J. Telling stories: exploring research storytelling as a meaningful approach to knowledge mobilization with Indigenous research collaborators and diverse audiences in community-based participatory research. Can Geogr 2012;56(2):231–42.
28. Haozous EA, Knobf MT. All my tears were gone: suffering and cancer pain in Southwest American Indians. J Pain Symptom Manage 2013;45(6):1050–60.
29. Hurst S, Nader P. Building community involvement in cross-cultural Indigenous health problems. Int J Qual Health Care 2006;184(4):294–8.
30. Begay RC. A women's shelter in a rural American Indian community. Fam Community Health 2011;34(3):229–34.
31. Shubair MM, Tobin PK. Type 2 diabetes in the First Nations population: a case example of clinical practice guidelines. Rural Remote Health 2010;10(1505):1–7.
32. Cross T. Relational worldview model. Pathways Practice Digest 1997;12(4). Available at: http://www.nicwa.org/relational_worldview/. Accessed January 29, 2015.
33. Vogel O, Cowens-Alvarado R, Eschiti V, et al. Circle of life cancer education: giving voice to American Indian and Alaska Native communities. J Cancer Educ 2013;28:565–72.
34. Kanekar S, Petereit D. Walking forward: a program designed to lower cancer mortality rates among American Indians in Western South Dakota. S D Med 2009; 62(4):151–9.
35. Andrews JO, Felton G, Wewers ME, et al. Use of community health workers in research with ethnic minority women. J Nurs Scholarsh 2004;36(4):358–65.
36. Haozous EA, Doorenbos AZ, Demiris G, et al. Role of telehealth/videoconferencing in managing cancer pain in rural American Indian communities. Psychooncology 2012;21(2):219–23.
37. Doorenbos AZ, Kundu A, Eaton LH, et al. Enhancing access to cancer education for rural healthcare providers via telehealth. J Cancer Educ 2011;26:682–6.

Enhancing the Collection, Discussion and Use of Family Health History by Consumers, Nurses and Other Health Care Providers

 CrossMark

Because Family Health History Matters

Sandra Millon Underwood, PhD, RN, FAAN[a],*, Sheryl Kelber, MA[b]

KEYWORDS

- Family health history • Genetics • Genomics • Personalized medicine

KEY POINTS

- The family health history is a powerful tool that can be used by health care providers to identify common diseases and rare diseases prevalent in families.
- Information from a patient's family health history can draw the attention of providers to red flags commonly associated with genetic risks and can be used to develop personalized preventive health care plans.
- Data highlighted in this report suggest the need for more targeted efforts by nurses and other health care providers to increase public awareness of the importance of family health history and to promote discussion about family health history among individuals and families. Data also suggest the need for similar efforts by leaders in the clinical and academic arena to review, reinforce, and reaffirm the value, importance, and relevance of the family health history among nurses and other health care providers in the practice setting.

This work was supported by the Wisconsin Department of Health and Family Services and the University of Wisconsin Milwaukee Undergraduate Research Program.
Conflicts of Interest: The authors have no conflicts of interest to report.
[a] University of Wisconsin Milwaukee College of Nursing, 1921 East Hartford, Milwaukee, WI 53211, USA; [b] Harriet H. Werley Center for Nursing Research and Evaluation, University of Wisconsin Milwaukee College of Nursing, 1921 East Hartford, Milwaukee, WI 53211, USA
* Corresponding author.
E-mail address: underwoo@uwm.edu

INTRODUCTION

Advances being made by genetic and genomic scientists domestically and abroad are impacting all facets of health care. Knowledge gleaned from genetic research is increasing the understanding of diseases that result from single-gene errors (eg, cystic fibrosis, sickle cell anemia, Huntington's disease, hereditary hemochromatosis, Tay-Sachs disease, glaucoma, Marfan syndrome, phenylketonuria). Knowledge gleaned from genomic research is, likewise, increasing the understanding of diseases caused by genetic mutations, lifestyle, and environmental factors (eg, heart disease, high blood pressure, Alzheimer's disease, Parkinson's disease, arthritis, diabetes, breast and colon cancer, and obesity/overweight). As a direct result, progress is being made relative to the identification of biomarkers of pathogenesis and the development of genetically based tools for use in the personalized assessment of health status and disease risk. Yet, in this era of genetics, genomics, and personalized health care, it is suggested that newly developed high-tech genetically based options do not completely overshadow low-tech tools currently used to assess a patient's health status and to evaluate their risk of both common and rare diseases. Rather they are reported to give them new meaning and power.

The family health history (FHH), often touted as the first genetic test administered in the health care setting, has been described by leaders in the field as "the most powerful genetic/genomic tool available to clinicians in general and specialized practice."[1–4] The FHH has long been used by nurses and other health care providers in clinical practice to determine if an individual, their family members, or their future generations are at an increased risk of heritable disease development (**Box 1**).[5,6] The FHH can reveal common diseases and rare diseases prevalent in families. The FHH can draw attention to red flags commonly associated with genetic risks, such as family history of multiple affected family members with the same disease or disorder; 2 or more generations of family members affected by the same disease; combinations of diseases within a family (eg, breast and ovarian cancer, heart disease and diabetes, diabetes and peripheral vascular disease); early onset of disease within a family (ie, onset of disease within a family 10–20 years before people are typically diagnosed); disease in the less-often-affected sex (eg, breast cancer in a male, persistent stuttering in a female); consecutive miscarriages, stillbirths, or sudden infant deaths; ethnic predisposition to genetic disorders (eg, sickle cell anemia or lactose intolerance in individuals of African ancestry, cystic fibrosis in whites of Northern European descent, BRCA 1/2 mutations and Tay-Sachs disease in individuals of Ashkenazi Jewish ancestry); and consanguinity (ie, children resulting from relationships between blood relatives who would be at an increased risk of having an autosomal recessive condition).[7,8] The FHH can similarly be used to identify social, environmental, and cultural factors that may impact an individual's health.

Several of reports in the peer-reviewed literature over the last decade address issues relevant to FHH. Included among them are reports that describe the origin and evolution of FHH[5,9–13]; reports that highlight the utility of FHH for identifying persons at risk of heritable disease development[14–19]; reports that describe patterns of communication and documentation of FHH common among diverse population groups[20–26]; and reports that delineate factors impacting the quality, quantity, and use of FHH in clinical practice.[27–29] Despite the expanding body of evidence substantiating the power of FHH as a genetic/genomic tool, the value of FHH for the assessment of disease risk, the importance of FHH to provision of health care in clinical practice, and the institution of national FHH campaigns by the Office of the United States Surgeon General[30] and the Centers for Disease Control and Prevention,[31]

| Box 1 |
| Common heritable diseases |
| Arthritis |
| Asthma |
| Cancer |
| Congenital defects |
| Cystic fibrosis |
| Diabetes mellitus |
| Down's syndrome |
| Glaucoma |
| Heart disease |
| Huntington's disease |
| Hypertension |
| Hypercholesteremia |
| Miscarriage, stillbirth, infertility |
| Muscular dystrophy |
| Peripheral vascular disease |
| Phenylketonuria |
| Pulmonary disorders |
| Polycystic kidney disease |
| Sickle cell disease |
| Stroke |
| Thalassemia |

few articles report surveillance efforts undertaken to examine the extent to which FHH is collected by those in the general public and the manner in which FHH is used by providers in clinical practice. An exploratory pilot study of the collection and use of FHH was therefore proposed. The study was designed to explore the extent to which FHH was collected by a targeted group of men and women, the extent to which health care providers discussed their health care risks with them based on their FHH, and the extent to which health care providers incorporated information from their FHH in their plan of care.

The organizing framework designed for the study included constructs from the Transtheoretical Model of Change and the Health Beliefs Model. The Transtheoretical Model of Change, an integrative biopsychosocial model originally developed DiClemente and Prochaska,[32,33] suggests that adoption of health behaviors is an intentional process of change involving thoughtful contemplation, preparation, and action. The Health Beliefs Model, a psychological model developed by social psychologists Hochbaum, Rosenstock, and Kegels,[34,35] suggests that a person's beliefs about health, perceived benefits to action, and cues/stimuli to act explain engagement (or lack of engagement) in a health-promoting behavior. The organizing framework hypothesized the influence of several individual and modifying factors on the collection, discussion, and use of FHH (**Fig. 1**). More specifically, the study framework hypothesized the influence of demographic, social, and economic factors; health concerns and

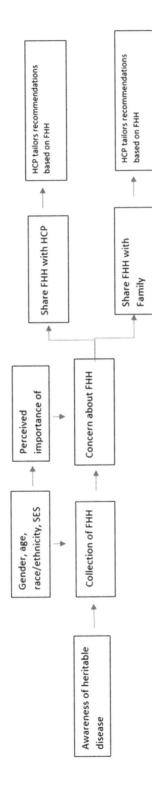

Fig. 1. Organizing framework.

perceptions relative to the importance of FHH; and family history of heritable diseases on the collection, discussion, and use of FHH. In applying the framework in this study, the dependent variables were the collection of FHH by patients, the discussion of FHH among patients and their health care providers, and the incorporation of information from the patient's FHH by the health care provider in the patient's plan of care. The independent variables were gender, age, marital status, parenting status, race/ethnicity, socioeconomic factors (ie, education, insurance status, primary care provider, and medical home), health concerns, perceptions relative to the importance of FHH, and family history of heritable diseases.

It was anticipated that the findings gleaned from the study would be relevant to nurses and other health care providers engaged in practices that emphasize health promotion and the management of health risks and to nurses and other health care providers whose practices focus on the prevention, diagnosis, and management of heritable diseases.

METHODS
Design

This cross-sectional study was designed to explore the collection, discussion and use of FHH among a targeted group of men and women who reside in the Midwestern United States.

Of particular interest was the influence of gender, age, marital status, parenting status, race/ethnicity, socioeconomic factors (ie, education, insurance status, primary care provider and medical home), health concerns, perceptions relative to the importance of FHH, and family history of heritable diseases on the collection of FHH among the study participants, the discussion of FHH by the study participants and their health care providers, and the incorporation of information from their FHH by health care providers in their plans of care.

Sample, Setting and Data Collection

A nonprobability sample of men and women from the general public was recruited to participate in the study. Prospective participants were 18 years of age and older, conversant in English, and willing to complete an FHH assessment survey. Study participants were recruited using proactive (face-to-face) recruitment methods at community centers, health centers, social service centers, and other public venues in urban and rural communities in the Midwestern United States. Before recruitment, the purpose of the study was described and the procedures to be used in gathering data were explained to the men and woman expressing an interest in participating in the study. An informed consent statement was presented and discussed with each prospective participant. Each prospective participant was informed that completion of the survey was voluntary and that receipt of services or support at the recruitment sites was not contingent on their participation. The prospective participants were informed that no names or personal identifiers would be requested or recorded. The men and women were informed that the information obtained from the study would be used to enhance the care provided to individuals and families within community-based and health care settings. Data were collected between June 1, 2014 and December 31, 2014.

Measures

An investigator-designed survey was constructed to collect the study data. The survey included measures used by the Centers for Disease Control and Prevention and state health departments to assess individual beliefs and practices regarding FHH and the use of FHH by HCPs.[36,37] Also included were measures designed to capture data reflective of the demographic, social, and economic characteristics; family health history; perceptions about the importance of FHH; and health concerns of the study participants.

Family history of heritable disease
Fourteen yes/no and contingency items were used to assess whether participants had a family history of asthma, cancer, diabetes, epilepsy, heart disease, glaucoma, hypertension, or sickle cell anemia. Participants who reported a family health history of asthma, cancer, diabetes, epilepsy, heart disease, glaucoma, hypertension, or sickle cell anemia were asked who in their immediate family had experienced the disease (ie, self, mother, father, sister, brother, children, grandmother, grandfather, aunt, uncle).

Perceived importance of family health history
One item was used to assess perceptions about the importance of FHH. Participants were asked to characterize their perceptions about the importance of FHH to their personal health using a 4-point Likert scale (eg, 1 = very important, 2 = somewhat important, 3 = not important at all, 4 = do not know).

Collection of family health history
Five yes/no contingency items were used to assess the collection of FHH. Participants were first asked if they had ever collected information from relatives for the purpose of developing an FHH. Participants who reported that they had collected information from relatives for the purpose of developing an FHH were asked if they shared the FHH information with their health care providers and family members.

Discussion and use of family health history by health care providers
Ten yes/no contingency items were used to assess the discussion and use of FHH by health care providers. Participants who reported that they had shared their FHH with their health care provider were asked if their "health care provider discussed their FHH" and if "health care provider made recommendations based on their FHH" (ie, dietary changes, exercise, weight management, smoking cessation, prescription medication, screening, genetic testing).

Perceived health concerns
One yes/no contingency item was used to assess perceived health concerns. Participants who reported a family health history of asthma, cancer, diabetes, epilepsy, heart disease, glaucoma, hypertension, or sickle cell anemia were asked if they were concerned about these diseases.

Demographic, social, and economic characteristics
Seventeen items were included in the survey to elicit data reflective of the participant's gender, age, marital status, parenting status, race/ethnicity and socioeconomic status (ie, education, insurance status, primary care provider, and medical home).

Validity, utility, and appropriateness of the survey for use among the targeted population were assessed by a panel of experts before initiation of the study.

Data Analysis

Descriptive and inferential statistics, computed using SPSS-PC Version 22 (SPSS Inc, Chicago, IL) were used to analyze the study data. Descriptive statistics (ie, frequency and percentages) were used to describe the characteristics of the study sample.

Inferential statistics (ie, cross tabulations, χ^2 analyses, odds ratios, and multiple logistic regression) were used to evaluate the influence of demographic, social, and economic factors; health concerns; perceived importance of FHH; and family history of heritable diseases on the collection, discussion, and use of FHH. A backwards elimination was used to determine the model with the best fit.

RESULTS
Participant Profile

A total of 709 men and women participated in the study (**Table 1**). Thirty-seven percent (n = 259) were men and 63.5% (n = 450) were women. Sixty-two percent (n = 437) reported their race/ethnicity as white, 17.3% (n = 123) reported black, 13.8% (n = 98) reported Hispanic, 2.1% (15) reported Asian, and 0.6% (n = 4) reported Native American. The age of the study participants ranged from 18 to 88 years (mean, 36.19; SD = 17.12). Fifty percent (n = 353) reported that they were married, partnered, divorced, separated, or widowed, and 48.9% (n = 347) reported their marital status as single/never married. Fifty percent (n = 357) reported that they were the parents of biological children. Sixty eight percent (n = 485) of the study participants reported having attended or graduated from college. Eighty-seven percent (n = 615) reported they were insured. Eighty-one percent (n = 576) reported that they had a primary health care provider. Fifty-five percent (n = 391) reported that they had a medical home where they routinely received medical care.

History of Heritable Disease

Ninety percent (n = 643) of the study participants reported a family history of asthma, cancer, diabetes, epilepsy, heart disease, glaucoma, hypertension, or sickle cell anemia. The most common heritable diseases reported were hypertension (67.3%, n = 477), cancer (65.6%, 461), diabetes (51.5%, n = 365), heart disease (49.4%, n = 359) and asthma (41.0%; n = 291). Among those reporting a family history of a heritable disease only 38.6% (n = 248) expressed a concern about their health status.

Given the known impact of first-, second-, and third-degree family history of disease on risk status, the first-degree family history of disease was similarly ascertained. Seventy-one percent (n = 501) of the study participants reported a first-degree family history of asthma, cancer, diabetes, epilepsy, heart disease, glaucoma, hypertension, or sickle cell anemia. The most common first degree heritable diseases reported were hypertension (49.8%, 353), cancer (30.2, n = 214), diabetes (27.8%, n = 197), heart disease (26.4%, n = 187), and asthma (11.8%, n = 84). Among those reporting a first-degree family history of heritable disease, 57.8% (n = 288) reported that they were not concerned about their health status.

Collection, Discussion and Use of Family Health History

Sixty percent (n = 424) of the study participants reported that they had collected information from their relatives for the purpose of developing an FHH. Fifty-two percent (n = 366) reported that they had shared the FHH information with their health care providers, 42.7% (n = 303) reported that their health care provider discussed their health risks with them based on their FHH, and 33.6% (n = 238) reported that their health care provider made recommendations for screening/diagnostic testing, dietary modification, exercise, or weight management based on their FHH.

Among study participants reporting a first-degree family history of a heritable disease, 64% (n = 319) indicted that they had collected information from their relatives

Table 1
Demographic profile of the study participants (N = 709)

Characteristics	Number of Respondents	%
Gender		
Male	259	36.5
Female	450	63.5
Age (y)		
<35	395	55.7
35 or older	314	44.3
Marital status		
Single, never married	347	48.9
Married	277	39.1
Partnered	16	2.3
Divorced	40	5.6
Separated	7	1.0
Widowed	13	1.8
Not reported	9	1.3
Parenting status		
Have biological children	357	50.4
Have no biological children	352	49.6
Race/ethnicity		
White, non-Hispanic	437	61.6
Black, non-Hispanic	123	17.3
Hispanic	98	13.8
Asian	15	2.1
Native American	4	0.6
Multi-racial/ethnic	12	1.7
Not reported	20	2.8
Education		
Less than high school degree	42	5.9
High school degree, GED	155	21.9
Some college	331	46.7
College degree or higher	154	21.7
Health insurance status		
Insured	615	86.7
Uninsured	94	13.3
Family history of heritable disease*		
First-, second-, or third-degree family history of heritable disease	644	90.8
First-degree family history of heritable disease	501	70.7
No reported family history of heritable disease	65	9.2
Concern about health status		
Yes	264	37.2
No	445	62.8

(continued on next page)

Table 1 (continued)		
Characteristics	Number of Respondents	%
Health care provider		
Yes	575	81.2
No	133	18.8
Medical home		
Yes	391	55.1
No	318	44.9
Perceived importance of FHH		
Very important	499	70.4
Somewhat important	177	25.0
Not important	23	3.2
I do not know	10	1.4

* Family history of heritable disease (asthma, cancer, diabetes, epilepsy, heart disease, glaucoma, hypertension, or sickle cell anemia).

and developed an FHH, 55.3% (n = 277) reported that they had shared the information with their health care providers, 46.1% (n = 231) reported that their health care provider discussed their health risks with them based on their FHH, and 37.3% (n = 187) reported that their health care provider made recommendations for screening/diagnostic testing, dietary changes, exercise, weight management, behavior modification, or prescription medications based on their FHH.

Factors Associated with the Collection, Discussion and Use of Family Health History

Analyses using χ^2 and multivariate logistic regression models were used to assess the influence of demographic, social, and economic factors; health concerns; perceived importance of FHH; and family history of heritable diseases on the collection, discussion, and use of FHH. Study findings implicate the influence of several of these factors on the collection, discussion, and use of FHH (**Tables 2–4**). For example, study participants who were female, white, non-Hispanic, and single, who perceived that FHH was important to their health status were more likely to report the collection of FHH than study participants who were male, minority, Hispanic, and not single, who did not perceive that FHH was important to their health status (χ^2 = 12.124, degrees of freedom [df] = 1, $P<.001$; χ^2 = 16.341, df = 1, $P<.001$; χ^2 = 24.106, df = 1, $P<.001$; χ^2 = 24.848, df = 2, $P<.001$, respectively). Study participants who were female, single, who had a health care provider, who expressed a concern about their health status, and who perceived that FHH was important to their health status were more likely to indicate that their health care provider made recommendations for screening/diagnostic testing, dietary changes, exercise, weight management, behavior modification, or prescription medications based on their FHH than participants who were male, single, who did have a health care provider, who did perceive that FHH was important to their health status (χ^2 = 6.933, df = 1, P = .008; χ^2 = 17.271, df = 1, $P<.001$; χ^2 = 16.018, df = 1, $P<.001$; χ^2 = 16.018 df = 1, $P<.001$; χ^2 = 21.976, df = 2, $P<.001$, respectively). Study participants who were female, single, who had a designated health care provider, who expressed a concern about their health status, and who perceived that FHH was important to their health status were noted to be more likely report that they had discussions with

Table 2
Influence of individual/modifying factors on the collection of FHH (N = 709)

	Reported Collection of FHH % (95% CI)	No Reported Collection of FHH % (95% CI)	χ^2	df	P Value
Gender			12.124	1	.000
Male	51.4 (47.72–55.08)	48.6 (44.92–52.28)			
Female	64.7 (61.18–68.22)	35.3 (31.78–38.82)			
Age (y)			3.551	1	.060
<35	56.7 (53.05–60.35)	43.3 (39.65–46.95)			
35 or older	63.7 (60.16–67.24)	36.3 (32.76–39.84)			
Marital status			21.711	5	.001
Single	55.0 (51.34–58.66)	45.0 (41.34–48.66)			
Married	70.0 (66.63–73.37)	30.0 (26.63–33.37)			
Partnered	43.8 (40.15–47.45)	56.3 (52.65–59.95)			
Divorced	50.0 (46.32–53.68)	50.0 (46.32–53.68)			
Separated	28.6 (25.27–31.93)	71.4 (68.07–74.73)			
Widowed	53.8 (50.13–57.47)	46.2 (42.53–49.87)			
Not reported	33.3(29.83–36.77)	66.7 (63.23–70.17)			
Parenting status			6.394	1	.011
Have biological children	35.6 (32.08–39.12)	64.4 (60.88–67.92)			
Have no biological children	44.9 (41.24–48.56)	55.1 (51.44–58.76)			
Race/ethnicity			28.223	5	.000
White, non-Hispanic	65.7 (62.21–69.19)	34.3 (30.81–37.79)			
Black, non-Hispanic	56.9 (53.25–60.55)	43.1 (39.45–46.75)			
Hispanic	37.8 (34.23–41.37)	62.2 (62.72–69.68)			
Asian	60.0 (56.39–63.61)	40.0 (36.39–43.61)			
Native American	50.0 (46.32–53.68)	50.0 (46.32–53.68)			
Multiracial/ethnic	41.7 (38.07–45.33)	58.7 (55.08–62.32)			
Education			28.453	3	.000
Less than high school degree	40.5 (36.89–44.11)	59.5 (55.89–63.11)			
High school degree, GED	61.3 (57.71–64.89)	38.7 (35.11–42.29)			
Some college	54.7 (51.04–58.36)	45.3 (41.64–48.96)			
College degree or higher	76.6 (73.48–79.72)	23.4 (20.28–26.52)			
Health insurance status			13.413	1	.000
Insured	62.4 (58.83–65.97)	37.6 (34.03–41.17)			
Uninsured	42.6 (38.96–46.24)	57.4 (53.76–61.04)			
Family history of heritable disease[a]			10.771	2	.005
Second- or third-degree family history of heritable disease	49.7 (46.02–53.38)	50.3 (46.62–53.98)			
First-degree family history of heritable disease	63.7 (60.16–67.24)	36.3 (32.76–39.84)			
No reported family history of heritable disease	52.3 (48.62–55.98)	47.7 (42.02–51.38)			
Health care provider			35.902	1	.000
Yes	65.1 (48.62–55.98)	34.9 (31.39–38.41)			
No	36.8 (33.25–40.35)	63.2 (59.65–66.75)			
Medical home			4.764	1	.029
Yes	63.4 (59.85–66.95)	36.6 (33.05–40.15)			
No	55.3 (51.64–58.96)	44.7 (41.04–48.36)			

(continued on next page)

	Reported Collection of FHH % (95% CI)	No Reported Collection of FHH % (95% CI)	χ^2	df	P Value
Table 2 *(continued)*					
Concern about health status			81.914	1	.000
Yes	81.4 (78.54–84.26)	18.6 (15.74–21.46)			
No	47.0 (43.33–50.67)	53.0 (49.33–56.67)			
Perceived importance of FHH			35.164	3	.000
Very important	65.7 (62.21–69.19)	34.3 (30.81–37.79)			
Somewhat important	50.3 (46.62–53.98)	49.7 (46.02–53.38)			
Not important	26.1 (22.87–29.33)	73.9 (70.67–77.13)			
I do not know	10.0 (7.79–12.21)	90.0 (87.79–92.21)			
	59.8 (56.19–63.41)	40.2 (36.69–43.81)			

[a] Before collapsing groups.

health care providers about their health risks than study participants who were male, single, who did not have a designated health care provider, who did not express a concern about their health status, and who did not perceive that FHH was important to their health status (χ^2 = 11.631, df = 1, P = . 001; χ^2 = 7.322, df = 1, P = .007; χ^2 = 29.310, df = 1, P<.001; χ^2 = ,183.139 df = 1, P<.001; χ^2 = 20.630, df = 3, P<.001).

Multivariate logistic regression models were used to assess the extent to which the demographic, social and economic factors, health concerns, perceived importance of FHH, and family history of heritable diseases predicted the collection, discussion and use of FHH. Age, gender, marital status, parenting status, race/ethnicity, socioeconomic factors (ie, education, insurance status, primary care provider and medical home), health concerns, perceptions relative to the importance of FHH, and family history of heritable diseases were entered into the logistic regression analysis as independent variables to be tested as predictive factors for collection, discussion and use of FHH. **Tables 5–7** show the results of the logistic regression analysis. Logistic regression analysis indicated that the model correctly predicted the collection of FHH of 66% of the study participants; correctly predicted the discussion of FHH of 76% of the study participants; and, correctly predicted the use of the FHH by healthcare providers of 79% of the study participants.

Discussion

The FHH has long been used by nurses and other health care providers in clinical practice to determine if an individual, their family members, or their future generations is/ are at an increased risk of developing heritable diseases.[5,6] The information gleaned from FHH has most often been used to make preliminary assessments of risk (**Fig. 2**), as a basis for planning screening and diagnostic testing, and to initiate plans of personalized health care (ie, health promotion, risk management, surveillance and treatment) (**Fig. 3**). Over the past decade, as research and health care progresses toward personalized healthcare, hundreds of high-tech genetically-based options for the assessment of health risks have been designed. Yet, amid the myriad options currently available, the FHH continues to be acclaimed by experts in the laboratory and in practice as the "gold standard" for the initial assessment of risk of common and rare diseases.

Numerous efforts have been launched by the United States Surgeon General[30] and the Centers for Disease Control and Prevention[31] to increase the public's

Table 3

Influence of individual/modifying factors on the discussion of FHH (N = 709)

	Reported Discussion of FHH with HCP % (95% CI)	No Reported Discussion of FHH with HCP % (95% CI)	χ^2	df	P Value
Gender			11.691	1	.001
Male	34.4 (30.90–37.90)	65.6 (62.1–69.1)			
Female	47.6 (43.92–51.28)	52.4 (48.72–58.08)			
Age (years)			8.263	1	.004
<35	38.0 (34.43–41.57)	62.0 (58.43–65.57)			
35 or older	48.7 (45.02–52.38)	51.3 (47.62–54.98)			
Marital status			15.224	6	.019
Single	37.8 (34.23–41.37)	62.2 (58.63–65.77)			
Married	50.5 (46.82–54.18)	49.5 (45.82–53.18)			
Partnered	18.8 (15.92–21.66)	81.3 (78.43–84.17)			
Divorced	45.0 (41.34–48.66)	55.0 (51.34–58.66)			
Separated	28.6 (25.27–31.93)	71.4 (68.07–74.73)			
Widowed	46.2 (42.53–49.87)	53.8 (50.13–57.47)			
Not reported	—	66.7 (63.23–70.17)			
Parenting status			7.832	1	.005
Have biological children	47.9 (44.22–51.58)	52.1 (48.42–55.78)			
Have no biological children	37.5 (33.94–41.06)	62.5 (58.94–66.06)			
Race/ethnicity			12.759	5	.026
White, non-Hispanic	47.1 (43.43–50.77)	52.9 (49.23–56.57)			
Black, non-Hispanic	39.0 (35.41–42.59)	61.0 (51.41–64.59)			
Hispanic	28.6 (25.27–31.93)	71.4 (68.07–74.73)			
Asian	40.0 (36.39–43.61)	60.0 (56.39–63.61)			
Native American	50.0 (46.32–53.68)	50.0 (46.32–53.68)			
Multiracial/ethnic	33.3 (29.83–36.77)	66.7 (63.23–70.17)			
Education			17.248	3	.001
Less than high school degree	31.0 (27.6–34.4)	69.0 (65.60–72.40)			
High school degree, GED	43.9 (40.25–47.55)	56.1 (52.45–59.75)			
Some college	38.1 (34.53–41.67)	61.9 (58.33–65.47)			
College degree or higher	56.5 (52.85–60.15)	43.5 (39.85–47.15)			

			χ²	df	P
Health insurance status			20.392	1	.000
Insured	46.0 (42.33–49.67)	54.0 (50.33–57.67)			
Uninsured	21.3 (18.29–24.31)	78.7 (75.69–81.71)			
Family history of heritable disease[a]			7.955	2	.019
Second- or third-degree family history of heritable disease	35.0 (31.49–38.51)	65.0 (61.49–68.51)			
First-degree family history of heritable disease	46.1 (42.43–49.77)	53.9 (50.23–57.57)			
No reported family history of heritable disease	33.8 (30.32–37.28)	66.2 (62.72–69.68)			
Health care provider			29.310	1	.000
Yes	47.6 (43.92–51.28)	52.4 (48.72–56.08)			
No	21.8 (18.76–24.84)	78.2 (75.16–81.24)			
Medical home			5.174	1	.023
Yes	46.5 (42.83–50.17)	53.5 (49.83–57.17)			
No	38.1 (34.53–41.67)	61.9 (58.33–65.47)			
Concern about health status			183.159	1	.000
Yes	75.4 (72.23–78.57)	24.6 (21.43–27.77)			
No	23.4 (20.28–26.52)	76.6 (73.48–79.72)			
Perceived importance of FHH			25.127	3	.000
Very important	48.5 (44.82–52.18)	51.5 (47.82–55.18)			
Somewhat important	31.1 (27.69–34.51)	68.9 (65.49–73.31)			
Not important	21.7 (18.67–24.73)	78.3 (75.27–81.33)			
I do not know	10.0 (7.79–12.21)	90.0 (87.79–92.21)			

Abbreviation: HCP, health care provider.
[a] Before collapsing groups.

Table 4
Influence of individual/modifying factors on recommendations made by HCP (N = 709)

	Recommendations Made by HCP	No Recommendations Made by HCP	χ^2	df	P Value
Gender			6.933	1	.008
Male	27.4 (24.12–30.68)	72.6 (69.32–75.88)			
Female	37.1 (33.54–40.66)	62.9 (59.34–66.46)			
Age (y)			19.520	1	.000
<35	26.6 (23.35–29.85)	73.4 (70.15–76.65)			
35 or older	42.4 (38.76–46.04)	57.6 (53.96–61.24)			
Marital status			22.722	6	.001
Single	26.2 (22.96–29.44)	73.8 (70.56–77.64)			
Married	43.0 (39.36–46.64)	57.0 (53.36–60.64)			
Partnered	18.8 (15.92–21.68)	81.3 (78.43–84.17)			
Divorced	37.5 (33.94–41.06)	62.5 (58.94–66.06)			
Separated	28.6 (25.27–31.93)	71.4 (68.07–74.73)			
Widowed	46.2 (25.27–31.93)	53.8 (50.13–57.47)			
Not reported	22.2 (19.14–25.26)	77.8 (74.74–80.86)			
Parenting status			16.017	1	.000
Have biological children	26.4 (23.16–29.64)	73.6 (74.74–80.86)			
Have no biological children	40.6 (39.99–44.21)	59.6 (55.99–63.21)			
Race/ethnicity			4.424	5	.490
White, non-Hispanic	35.9 (32.37–39.43)	64.1 (60.57–67.63)			
Black, non-Hispanic	30.1 (26.72–33.48)	69.9 (66.52–73.28)			
Hispanic	26.5 (23.25–29.75)	73.5 (70.25–76.75)			
Asian	33.3 (29.83–36.77)	66.7 (63.25–70.17)			
Native American	50.0 (46.32–53.68)	50.0 (46.32–53.68)			
Multiracial/ethnic	33.0 (29.54–36.46)	66.7 (63.23–70.17)			
	33.5 (30.03–36.97)	66.5 (63.03–69.97)			
Education			15.894	3	.001
Less than high school degree	28.6 (25.27–31.93)	71.4 (68.07–74.73)			
High school degree, GED	33.5 (30.03–36.97)	66.5 (63.03–69.97)			
Some college	28.7 (25.37–32.03)	71.3 (67.97–74.63)			
College degree or higher	46.8 (43.13–50.47)	53.2 (49.53–56.87)			
Health insurance status			7.342	1	.007
Insured	35.4 (31.88–38.92)	64.6 (61.08–68.12)			
Uninsured	21.3 (18.29–24.31)	78.7 (75.69–81.71)			
Family history of heritable disease[a]			10.809	2	.004
Second- or third-degree family history of heritable disease	24.5 (21.33–27.67)	75.5 (72.33–78.67)			
First-degree family history of heritable disease	37.3 (33.74–40.86)	62.7 (59.14–66.26)			
No reported family history of heritable disease	24.6 (21.43–27.77)	75.4 (72.23–78.57)			
Health care provider			16.018	1	.000
Yes	37.0 (33.45–40.55)	63.0 (59.45–66.55)			
No	18.8 (15.92–21.68)	81.2 (78.32–84.08)			

(continued on next page)

Table 4
(continued)

	Recommendations Made by HCP	No Recommendations Made by HCP	χ^2	df	P Value
Medical home			2.954	1	.086
Yes	36.3 (32.76–39.84)	63.7 (60.16–67.24)			
No	30.2 (26.82–33.58)	69.8 (66.42-73–18)			
Concern about health status			201.928	1	.000
Yes	66.3 (62.82–69.78)	33.7 (30.22–37.18)			
No	14.2 (11.63–16.77)	85.8 (83.23–88.37)			
Perceived importance of FHH			27.254	3	.000
Very important	39.3 (35.70–42.90)	60.7 (57.10–64.30)			
Somewhat important	22.0 (18.95–25.05)	78.0 (74.95–81.05)			
Not important	13.0 (10.52–15.48)	87.0 (84.52–89.48)			

Abbreviation: HCP, health care provider.
[a] Before collapsing groups.

awareness of the importance of FHH and to promote discussion about FHH among in communities and in the healthcare setting. The same of true of efforts undertaken by the National Human Genome Research Institute[38] and the American Society of Human Genetics[39] to enhance the integration of FHH by healthcare providers in practice. However, data from this study suggest a need for efforts to reaffirm the

Table 5
Logistic regression models for factors influencing collection of FHH (N = 709)

Factors	Number of Respondents	Number Reporting Collection of FHH	%	Odds Ratio	95% CI
Gender				1.57	(1.085–2.269)
Male	259	133	51		
Female	450	291	65		
Marital status				1.50	(1.050–2.142)
Single	353	230	65		
Not single	353	191	55		
Race/ethnicity				0.639	(0.440–0.927)
White, non-Hispanic	437	150	34		
Minority	272	35	50		
Health care provider				2.182	(1.388–3.431)
Yes	545	357	66		
No	164	67	41		
Concern about health status				4.329	(2.916–6.331)
Yes	264	215	81		
No	445	209	47		
Perceived importance of FHH				Reference	
Very important	499	328	66	0.0588	(0.391–0.883)
Somewhat important	177	89	50	0.247	(0.084–0.725)
Not important	23	6	26	0.116	(0.012–1.128)
I do not know	10	1	10	—	—

The overall percentage predicted from the model is 66%.
   The model correctly predicted 73% of the participants reporting collection of FHH and 55% of the participants reporting that they had not collected FHH.

Table 6
Logistic regression models for factors influencing discussion of FHH (N = 709)

Factors	Number of Respondents	Number Reporting Collection of FHH	%	Odds Ratio	95% CI
Gender				1.698	(1.131–2.548)
Male	259	89	34		
Female	450	214	48		
Marital status				1.489	(1.023–2.154)
Single	353	169	48		
Not single	353	131	38		
Health care provider				2.6	(1.513–4.417)
Yes	545	264	48		
No	164	39	24		
Concern about health status				9.598	(6.398–12.869)
Yes	264	199	75		
No	445	104	23		
Perceived importance of FHH				Reference	
Very important	499	242	49	0.598	(0.337–0.925)
Somewhat important	177	55	31	0.482	(0.132–1.648)
Not important	23	5	22	0.291	(0.024–3.288)
I do not know	10	1	10	—	—

The overall percentage predicted from the model is 76%.
The model correctly predicted 65% of the participants reporting discussion of FHH and 85% of the participants reporting that they had not discussed their FHH with their HCP.

Table 7
Logistic regression models for factors influencing recommendations made by health care provider based on the FHH (N = 709)

Factors	Number of Respondents	Number Reporting Collection of FHH	%	Odds Ratio	95% CI
Gender				1.601	(1.045–2.452)
Male	259	71	27		
Female	450	167	37		
Marital status				2.084	(1.396–3.111)
Single	353	145	41		
Not single	353	91	26		
Concern about health status				10.969	(7.424–15.951)
Yes	264	175	66		
No	445	63	14		
Perceived Importance of FHH				Reference	
Very important	499	196	39	0.498	(0.308–0.805)
Somewhat important	177	39	22	0.181	(0.071–0.134)
Not important	23	3	13	0	—
I do not know	10	0	0	—	—
Health care provider				1.806	(1.023–3.109)
Yes	545	264	48		
No	164	39	24		

The overall percentage predicted from the model is 79%.
The model correctly predicted 72% of the participants reporting that their health care provider made recommendations based on their FHH and 83% of the participants reporting that health care providers had not made recommendations based on their FHH.

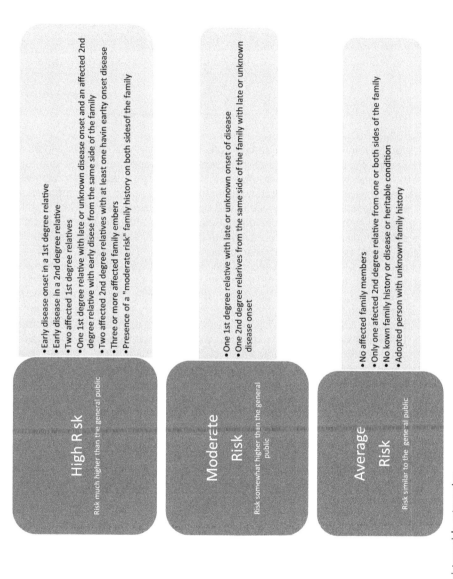

High Risk
Risk much higher than the general public

- Early disease onset in a 1st degree relative
- Early disease in a 2nd degree relative
- Two affected 1st degree relatives
- One 1st degree relative with late or unknown disease onset and an affected 2nd degree relative with early disese from the same side of the family
- Two affected 2nd degree relatives with at least one havin earlty onset disease
- Three or more affected family embers
- Presence of a "moderate risk" family history on both sidesof the family

Moderate Risk
Risk somewhat higher than the general public

- One 1st degree relative with late or unknown onset of disease
- One 2nd degree relatives from the same side of the family with late or unknown disease onset

Average Risk
Risk similar to the general public

- No affected family members
- Only one afected 2nd degree relative from one or both sides of the family
- No kown family history or disease or heritable condition
- Adopted person with unknown family history

Fig. 2. Family history risk categories.

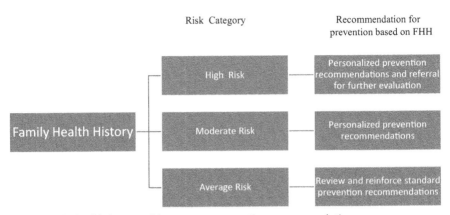

Fig. 3. Family health history, risk category, prevention recommendations.

importance and relevance of FHH among nurses and other healthcare providers in clinical practice. Findings from this study, much like those reported by Foland and Burke (2014)[40] and Yoon, Scheuner, Gwinn, & Khoury (2004),[41] suggest a relatively high level of knowledge and understanding in the general public of the importance of FHH, show deficits and differences in the collection of and use of FHH among men and women in the targeted population. Results of this study revealed that while the 95% of the study respondents believed that their family health history was important to their overall health, only 60% had collected health information from their relatives to develop an FHH, and 52% shared their FHH with their health care providers. Deficits in the collection and use of FHH were noted to be significantly lower among younger, unmarried, minority and uninsured. Similar deficits and differences were noted among participants with a first degree family history of a heritable disease. Among those with a first degree family history of a heritable disease 70%% reported that they believed that their family health history was important to their overall health, 64% reported collecting FHH, yet only 42% of those reporting a first degree history of a heritable disease reported sharing information from their FHH with their providers.

The FHH is a powerful tool that can be used by healthcare providers to identify common diseases and rare diseases prevalent in families. Information from the patient's FHH can also draw the attention of providers to "red flags" commonly associated with genetic risks. Healthcare providers can use and integrate and apply information gleaned from the FHH into their patient's plan of care in a number of ways. Most important would be the use of the information as a measure of health status, disease risk and, as a basis for initiating a personalized plan for personalized preventive health care (see **Figs. 2** and **3**).

Much effort has been undertaken over the past decade to increase the discussion, collection and compilation of FHHs by individuals and families in the general public. Yet, results from this study revealed that most participants had not engaged in discussions with their healthcare providers about their FHH. Data suggest the need for more targeted efforts by nurses and other healthcare providers to increase public awareness of the importance of FHH and to promote discussion about FHH among individuals and families. Data also suggest the need for similar efforts by leaders in the clinical and academic arena to review, reinforce and reaffirm the value, importance and relevance of the FHH among nurses and other health care providers in the practice setting.

> **Web tools and resources for nurses and other related healthcare providers**
>
> - American Association of Colleges of Nursing Genetic and Genomic Nursing Competencies—http://www.aacn.nche.edu/education-resources/Genetics__Genomics_Nursing_Competencies_09-22-06.pdf
> - American Society of Human Genetics: Family Health History Campaign—http://www.talkhealthhistory.org/
> - American Society of Human Genetics: Tools and Resources for Healthcare Providers—http://www.talkhealthhistory.org/healthcare/tools.shtml
> - American Society for Human Genetics: Tools and Resources for Families—http://www.talkhealthhistory.org/family/tools.shtml
> - Centers for Disease Control, Office of Genetics and Disease Prevention, Family History Public Health Initiative—http://www.cdc.gov/genomics/famhistory/
> - Genetic Alliance Health Provider Genetics Resources—http://geneticalliance.org/programs/genesinlife/fhh
> - US Surgeon General Family History Initiative—http://www.hhs.gov/familyhistory/
> - National Institutes of Health Promoting Family Health Initiative—http://nihseniorhealth.gov/creatingafamilyhealthhistory/promotingfamilyhealth/01.html

ACKNOWLEDGMENTS

The authors thank Gary Jechorek, University of Wisconsin Milwaukee, College of Nursing, Program Associate, for providing assistance and support with project implementation and data management.

REFERENCES

1. Yoon PW, Scheuner MT, Peterson-Oehlke KL, et al. Can family history be used as a tool for public health and preventive medicine? Genet Med 2002;4:304–10.
2. Beery TA, Shooner KA. Family history: the first genetic screen. Nurse Pract 2004; 29(11):14–25.
3. Wolpert CM, Speer MC. Harnessing the power of the pedigree. J Midwifery Womens Health 2005;50(3):189–96.
4. Maradiegue A, Edwards QT. An overview of ethnicity and assessment of family history in primary care settings. J Am Acad Nurse Pract 2006;18(10):447–56.
5. Pyeritz RE. The family history: the first genetic test, and still useful after all those years? Genet Med 2012;14(1):3–9.
6. Bancroft E, Ardern-Jones A, Lynch E. Cancer genetics: the importance of obtaining a family history. Nurs Times 2006;102(40):28–9.
7. Genetics in Primary Care Institute, 2015 Genetic red flags. Available at: http://www.geneticsinprimarycare.org/YourPractice/Family-HealthHistory/Pages/Genetic%20Red%20Flags.aspx. Accessed April 3, 2015.
8. Whelan AJ, Ball S, Best L, et al. Genetic red flags: clues to thinking genetically in primary care practice. Prim Care 2004;31(3):497–508.
9. Hinton RB. The family history: reemergence of an established tool. Crit Care Nurs Clin North Am 2008;20(2):149–58.
10. Kelly P. The importance of documenting family history. Crit Care Nurse 2011;31(4):18.
11. Alspach JG. The importance of family health history: your patients' and your own. Crit Care Nurse 2011;31(1):10–5.

12. Guttmacher AE, Collins FS, Carmona RH. The family history–more important than ever. N Engl J Med 2004;351(22):2333–6.
13. Bennett RL. The family medical history. Prim Care 2004;31(3):479–95.
14. Hanson C, Novilla L, Barnes M, et al. Using family health history for chronic disease prevention in the age of genomics: translation to health education practice. Am J Health Educ 2007;38(4):219–29.
15. Feiero WG, Bigley MB, Brinner KM, Family Health History Multi-Stakeholder Workgroup of the American Health Information Community. New standards and enhanced utility for family health history information in the electronic health record: an update from the American Health Information Community's Family Health History Multi-Stakeholder Workgroup. J Am Med Inform Assoc 2008;15(6):723–8.
16. Vogel KJ, Murthy VS, Dudley B, et al. The use of family health histories to address health disparities in an African American community. Health Promot Pract 2007; 8(4):350–7.
17. Yoon PW, Scheuner MT, Jorgensen C, et al. Developing Family Healthware, a family history screening tool to prevent common chronic diseases. Prev Chronic Dis 2009;6(1):A33.
18. Murray MF, Giovanni MA, Klinger E, et al. Comparing electronic health record portals to obtain patient-entered family health history in primary care. J Gen Intern Med 2013;28(12):1558–64.
19. Murthy VS, Garza MA, Almario DA, et al. Using a family history intervention to improve cancer risk perception in a black community. J Genet Couns 2011; 20(6):639–49.
20. Corona R, Rodríguez V, Quillin J, et al. Talking (or not) about family health history in families of Latino young adults. Health Educ Behav 2013;40(5):571–80.
21. Kaphingst KA, Goodman M, Pandya C, et al. Factors affecting frequency of communication about family health history with family members and doctors in a medically underserved population. Patient Educ Couns 2012;88(2):291–7.
22. Ashida S, Kaphingst KA, Goodman M, et al. Family health history communication networks of older adults: importance of social relationships and disease perceptions. Health Educ Behav 2013;40(5):612–9.
23. Thompson T, Seo J, Griffith J, et al. "You don't have to keep everything on paper": African American women's use of family health history tools. J Community Genet 2013;4(2):251–61.
24. Ashida S, Schafer EJ. Family health information sharing among older adults: reaching more family members. J Community Genet 2015;6(1):17–27.
25. Molster C, Kyne G, O'Leary P. Motivating intentions to adopt risk-reducing behaviors for chronic diseases: impact of a public health tool for collecting family health histories. Health Promot J Austr 2011;22(1):57–62.
26. Koehly LM, Ashida S, Goergen AF, et al. Willingness of Mexican-American adults to share family health history with healthcare providers. Am J Prev Med 2011; 40(6):633–6.
27. Hartmann CD, Marshall PA, Goldenberg AJ. Is there a space for place in family history assessment? Underserved community views on the impact of neighborhood factors on health and prevention. J Prim Prev 2015;36(2):119–30.
28. Hovick SR, Yamasaki JS, Burton-Chase AM, et al. Patterns of family health history communication among older African American adults. J Health Commun 2015; 20(1):80–7.
29. Yamasaki J, Hovick SR. "That was grown folks' business": narrative reflection and response in older adults' family health history communication. Health Commun 2015;30(3):221–30.

30. Surgeon General's Family Health History Initiative. Available at: http://www.hhs. gov/familyhistory/. Accessed April 3, 2015.
31. Centers for Disease Control Family History Public Health Initiative. Available at: http://www.cdc.gov/genomics/famhistory/. Accessed April 3, 2015.
32. DiClemente CC. Changing addictive behaviors: a process perspective. Curr Dir Psychol Sci 1993;2:101–6.
33. DiClemente C, Prochaska J. Toward a comprehensive, transtheoretical model of change. In: Miller W, Heather N, editors. Treating addictive behaviours. New York: Plenum Press; 1998. p. 3–27.
34. Rosenstock I. Historical origins of the health belief model. Health Educ Monogr 1974;2(4):328–35.
35. Stretcher VJ, Rosenstock IM. The health belief model. San Francisco (CA): JosseyBass; 1997.
36. Centers for Disease Control and Prevention. Behavioral risk factor surveillance system survey questionnaire. Atlanta (GA): U.S. Department of Health and Human Services, Centers for Disease Control and Prevention; 2014. Available at: http://www.cdc.gov/brfss/questionnaires.htm.
37. University of Washington Center for Genomics & Public Health. 2011. Family history and genomics questions from state-added BRFSS modules. 2011. Available at: http://depts.washington.edu/cgph/pdf/Static_BRFSS_Compilation.pdf. Accessed April 3, 2015.
38. National Human Genome Research Institute. Available at: https://www.genome. gov/. Accessed April 3, 2015.
39. American Society of Human Genetics. Understanding Genetics: A Guide for Patients and Health Professionals. Available at: http://www.geneticalliance.org/ publications/understandinggenetics. Accessed April 14, 2015.
40. Foland J, Burke B. Family health history data collection in Connecticut. Hartford (CT): Connecticut Department of Public Health, Genomics Office; 2014. Available at: http://www.ct.gov/dph/lib/dph/genomics/FHH_Brief_2014.pdf. Accessed April 14, 2015.
41. Yoon PW, ScD, Scheuner MT, MD, Gwinn M, MD, Khoury MJ, MD, PhD, Office of Genomics and Disease Prevention; Jorgensen C, DrPH, Div of Cancer Prevention and Control, National Center for Chronic Disease Prevention and Health Promotion; Hariri S, PhD, Lyn S, MD, EIS officers, CDC. Available at: http://www.cdc. gov/mmwr/preview/mmwrhtml/mm5344a5.htm. Accessed April 14, 2015.

Health Information Seeking Among Rural African Americans, Caucasians, and Hispanics: It Is Built, Did They Come?

Barbara D. Powe, PhD, RN, FAAN

KEYWORDS

- Health information seeking • Digital divide • Rural disparities • Social media
- Internet access and devices

KEY POINTS

- Socioeconomic disparities exist among rural populations of African Americans, Caucasians, and Hispanics that mirror the general population.
- Rural African Americans, Caucasians, and Hispanics do not seek health information at high rates.
- Rural African Americans, Caucasians, and Hispanics have access to the Internet but do not typically use it as a source of health information.
- Traditional sources of information such printed materials, television, and radio should be incorporated with Internet sources to provide a multiplatform approach for health information sharing.
- More research is needed to address health literacy, numeracy, navigation of Web sites, and strategies to establish trustworthiness of the information to facilitate the use of these resources by rural populations.

INTRODUCTION

Health information seeking refers to the act of searching for or gathering information and receiving messages that may be helpful in reducing uncertainty about health status and constructing a social and personal sense of health. It includes "any non-routine media use or interpersonal conversation about a specific health topic and thus includes behaviors such as viewing a special program about a health-related

Disclosures: This research was funded by the American Cancer Society (Intramural). The author has no financial or other conflicts of interest to report.
Lilburn, GA 30047, USA
E-mail address: pbarbd@comcast.net

Nurs Clin N Am 50 (2015) 531–543
http://dx.doi.org/10.1016/j.cnur.2015.05.007
0029-6465/15/$ – see front matter © 2015 Elsevier Inc. All rights reserved.

treatment, using a search engine to find information about a particular health topic on the Internet, and/or posing specific health-related questions to a friend, family member, or medical provider outside the normal flow of conversation."[1] In recent years, institutions such as bookstores, magazines, newspapers, and publishers of printed materials have been replaced or downsized because of the vast resources of and quick access to information that is available via the Internet. The growth of the Internet has also changed how public health organizations relay health information to constituents. In the past, 1-800 phone numbers, brochures, mail, and one-on-one conversations were common strategies used to provide information to the public. Although these strategies are still used to a lesser degree, it is much more common to see information placed on Web sites, which means the information can be changed or updated quickly and constituents have almost immediate access to it. As the Internet, as a public health tool, grew in popularity, the issue of the digital divide was raised. The digital divide referred to the fact that many, particularly those who were poor and underserved, did not have access to computers and software and thus were not able to access the resources on the Internet. Therefore, this lack of access was believed to create greater disparities in the provision of health care services, leading to poorer outcomes as well as higher mortality rates for the poor and underserved. As the cost of computers decreased over time and technologies such as smartphones and tablets become affordable options that could be used to access the Internet, it was initially believed that the digital divide was getting smaller.[2] However, this is not the case. The initial digital divide has now been replaced with what is referred to as a second-level digital divide or usage gap defined as differences in how many such as social and racial/ethnic groups use the Internet.[3] Specifically, people differ in their abilities to use the devices, their ability to navigate the online environments, their ability to determine trustworthy information online, and digital literacy (ability to understand and interpret the information).[4,5] Further, with the prevalence of the Internet, there are unanswered questions about how traditional media (print, television, radio, family, provider) are or are not used for health information in the technological age.[6]

Nurses are often seen as experts in providing patient education across the care continuum (prevention through treatment, cure, and survivorship). However, with changes in how the public access health care coupled with the availability of information and resources via the Internet, patients must now assume a greater role in independently seeking health information as opposed to waiting for it to be provided to them by nurses or other health care providers. Nurses as well as those directly responsible for publishing information in the online environment should be aware of the characteristics of those seeking information to ensure the information is placed using the right online platform (eg, social media vs Web site), can be accessed using the preferred device (eg, smartphone vs computer), and the information targets specific demographics, if appropriate. Research suggests that those who actively seek health information tend to be younger, Caucasian, and female and have higher incomes, higher education, and a usual source of care.[7–11] However, these characteristics highlight that those who are older, have lower incomes, have less education, and represent minority groups are less likely to seek health information. Specifically, it is known that there are differences in socioeconomic status, access to care, and access to information between urban and rural populations.[5,12,13] This fact is critical because these characteristics also describe those who have higher incidence and mortality rates from diseases such as diabetes, cancer, and cardiovascular disease. Therefore, the lack of access to health information has the potential to further widen the disparities gap for historically poor and underserved populations. Yet, few nurse-led studies have focused on the health-seeking behaviors among those who are rural, are racially/ethnically diverse, and may have decreased socioeconomic status. This information is important as this population represents a cross section of the American population, and studies that focus on race/ethnicity, geography, or socio-economic status in isolation may miss the complex interrelationships among these variables that influence health care from prevention to treatment and survival. The current descriptive, cross-sectional study focuses on the issue of race/ethnicity within the context of geography by addressing the following questions.

1. What sources do rural African American, Caucasians, and Hispanics use to seek health information?
2. What are the similarities and differences in access to technology among rural African Americans, Caucasians, and Hispanics?
3. What are the similarities and differences in online (Internet) activities among rural African Americans, Caucasians, and Hispanics?

METHODS
Sample and Setting

This study is part of a larger study that examined health-seeking behaviors across strata, race/ethnicity, age, income, education, and geography in California, Georgia, and Maryland. Because we were interested in looking at health-seeking behaviors across different demographic variables, we used a quota sampling strategy. This strategy allowed us to recruit participants based on demographics (race/ethnicity, age, education, income, geography) so that we had sufficient numbers to perform statistical analyses. Our sample was selected from a sampling frame of 20,000 individuals from California, Georgia, and Maryland so that we had access to diverse populations who would meet the study criteria for the quota sampling. Further, to reach the sample, we used the GENESYS Sampling System,[14] which included a database consisting of most residential telephone numbers and working cell phone numbers within the targeted geographic areas (California, Georgia, Maryland).

Surveys

The data collection survey was developed by the researchers using a combination of investigator-generated questions and standardized questions from the Health Information and National Trends Survey[15] and Pew Foundation Surveys.[16] The comprehensive survey used questions to collect data in 7 categories. These categories were (1) demographic information, (2) quality of life, (3) personal and family history of cancer, (4) cancer screening and early detection behaviors, (5) health information–seeking behaviors and sources used, (6) use of printed and mass media, and (7) use of the Internet, mobile technology, and social media platforms. There was a mixture of response sets based on the questions. For example, participants answered yes or no to whether they had insurance and were given a response set when choosing the type of insurance they had. These types of questions also allowed an other response in which the participant provided the information to the interviewer. Participants were asked to identify the frequency of behaviors such as how often they access the Internet using a predefined response set such as 1 to 2 hours per day, 3 to 4 hours per day, ending with more than 6 hours per day. Lastly, there were interval responses in which participants were asked how many hours they participated in an activity. For example, they were asked how many hours per day they watched television. The mixture of response sets allowed the researcher to gain a more comprehensive view of specific behaviors within and across the 7 questionnaire categories.

Procedures

The study was approved by the Institutional Review Board of Emory University (Atlanta, GA, USA). Interviews were completed by phone (landline, 67%, and cell phone, 33%). Interviews were conducted by trained data collectors employed by the company called the Independent Data Collection Center (Gainesville, FL, USA).[17] It was important to standardize the procedures for how the data collectors contacted the study participants by phone, read the survey, and marked the appropriate answers. Therefore, the data collectors used a computer-assisted telephone interviewing (CATI) system. The CATI system is a technique in which the interviewer follows a script provided by a software application.[18] The CATI system and script were pilot tested and revisions made as needed. The data collectors were trained on the study protocol with quality control monitors to ensure consistency across the interviews. There were protocols to address issues such as unanswered phones, voice mail, and participant refusals.

On average, the interviews were completed in 15 minutes, and participants received a $10 gift card by mail for their participation.

RESULTS
Demographics

The sample (N = 471) included African American (26%), Caucasian (46%), and Hispanic (28%) participants from rural areas of California (32%), Georgia (39%), and Maryland (29%). Most of the sample reported their overall health status as good or very good, with younger participants reporting better health. Those aged 20 to 39 years were more likely to report having good or very good health compared with other age groups. More Caucasians (19%) reported a personal diagnosis of cancer and were more likely to report a family history of cancer (65%) compared with African Americans (54%) and Hispanics (41%). Most of the participants in the sample were women and between the ages of 40 and 64 years, but Hispanics tended to be younger, whereas African Americans tended to be the older of the groups. African Americans and Hispanics had lower levels of education than Caucasians, who were also more likely to have private insurance compared with no insurance or Medicaid/Medicare. The majority (66%) of Caucasians had annual incomes greater than $20,000. Lastly, Hispanics were more likely to be married than African Americans and Caucasians.

Sources Rural African American, Caucasians, and Hispanics Use to Seek Health Information

Less than half of the sample reported having *ever* looked for information on health and/or medical topics from any source (**Fig. 1**). Of those who had looked for health or medical information, the Internet and the physician/health care provider were the most common sources used. Printed sources (books, brochures, magazines) were used as information sources (**Fig. 2**). Caucasians were more likely to report using family as an information source. On average, the participants watched television (TV) 3.59 hours per day and listened to the radio 2.19 hours per day. Although African Americans reported watching more TV, the groups did not report TV as a primary source of health information. Of the small number of participants reporting cancer organizations as an information source, Caucasians were more likely to use this resource ($df=2$, $\chi^2=6.94$, $P=.03$).

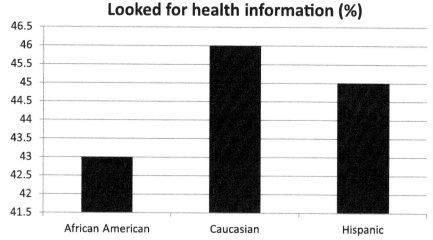

Fig. 1. Participants who sought health information in the past 12 months by race/ethnicity.

Similarities and Differences in Access to Technology Among Rural African Americans, Caucasians, and Hispanics

Participants were asked several questions about their phone service (**Fig. 3**). Less than 40% of the sample reported having a smartphone of any type. African Americans and Caucasians were more likely to have a basic cell phone (nonsmartphone) than Hispanics ($df=2, \chi^2=7.10, P=.03$). African Americans and Hispanics were more likely to have a landline than Caucasians ($df=2, \chi^2=26.0, P<.0001$). Less than 20% of participants had an iPad[19] or other type of tablet device. Although only approaching statistically significant values ($P = .07$), Caucasians were more likely to have a desktop (42%) and/or laptop (48%) computer than African Americans (32% and 40%, respectively) and Hispanics (36% and 32%, respectively). Caucasians (73%) were significantly more likely to report regular access to the Internet (ability to use it at any

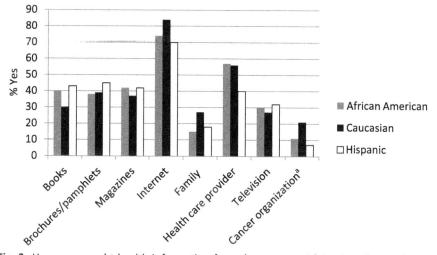

Fig. 2. Have you sought health information from these sources? [a] Statistically significant.

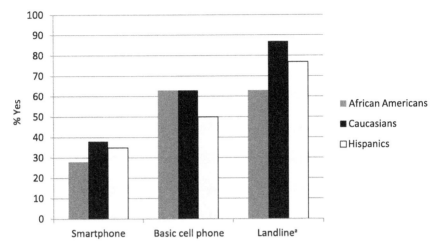

Fig. 3. Do you have these phones? [a] Statistically significant.

time) than African Americans (53%) or Hispanics (50%) ($df=2, \chi^2=22.86, P<.0001$). Most of the participants accessed the Internet via a broadband cable connection or dial-up system in their homes. Although not statistically significant, about 24% of Caucasians and 24% of Hispanics reported using their smartphone to access the Internet compared with 8% of African Americans. African Americans and Caucasians spent about 4 hours per day using the Internet for personal (non–work related) reasons compared with about 2 hours for Hispanics ($df=2$, $F=1.35, P=.261$).

Similarities and Differences in Online (Internet) Activities Among Rural African Americans, Caucasians, and Hispanics

Most participants sent and received e-mails using the Internet and received texts on the phone, but few had ever downloaded an application (app) to track or monitor their health (**Fig. 4**). Participants were asked if they read health-related pop-up messages

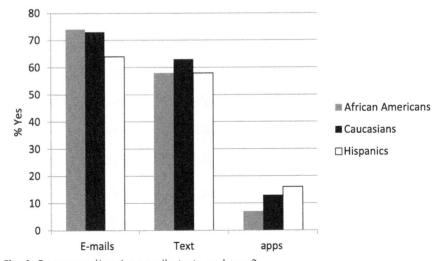

Fig. 4. Do you send/receive e-mails, texts, and apps?

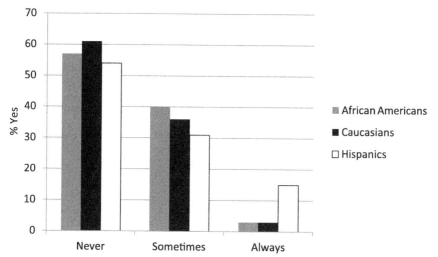

Fig. 5. Do you read health-related pop-up messages on the Internet?

while they were using the Internet. Although most of the sample responded that they "never" read them, more African Americans and Caucasians reported they "sometimes" read pop-up messages (**Fig. 5**). Most participants reported some level of trust of Web sites that provided health information (**Fig. 6**). However, only 25% of the sample would want their health care provider to send them information on their health by e-mail.

Caucasians (59%) and Hispanics (51%) were more likely to have visited a social networking site within the past 12 months than African Americans (42%) ($df=2, \chi^2=6.0, P=.05$). Most participants created personal profiles on Facebook[20] but less so on other social networking sites and reported an average of 215 friends

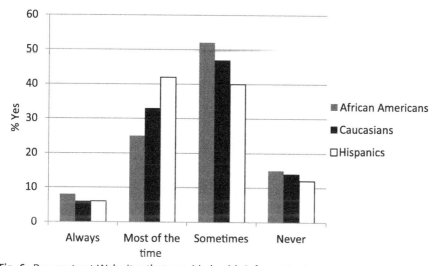

Fig. 6. Do you trust Web sites that provide health information?

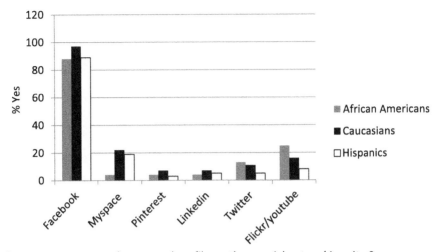

Fig. 7. Have you created a personal profile on these social networking sites?

in their network (**Figs. 7** and **8**). Most participants used the social networking sites to keep in touch with family and friends and share pictures but were less likely to use it to make professional contacts or meet new people (**Fig. 9**). Caucasians spent an average of 7 hours per week on social networking sites compared with Hispanics (5.8 hours) and African Americans (4.8 hours). Less than 6% of the sample had posted an online Weblog (blog). Less than 20% had used an online support group or looked for persons who had similar health conditions.

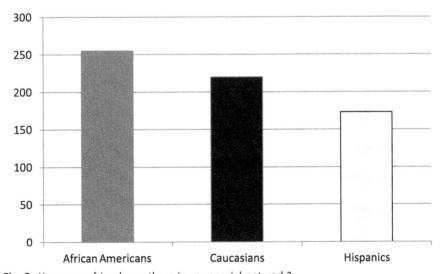

Fig. 8. How many friends are there in your social network?

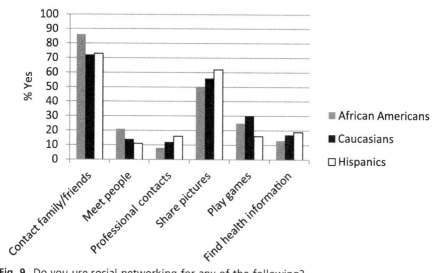

Fig. 9. Do you use social networking for any of the following?

DISCUSSION

Leading monitoring and evaluation groups continually provide updates, indicators, and predictions on how Americans access and use technology.[15,16] Leading indicators have acknowledged the gap or disparity in access and usage of technology based on race/ethnicity, gender, income, education, and living in an urban versus rural location.[4,21] Yet few, if any, empirical nurse-led studies have addressed health information–seeking behaviors and access to technology among rural populations as a specific subgroup. The consideration of similarities and differences across race/ethnicity within the context of rural populations is important because, although there is a culture of rurality, there is also a culture associated with the race/ethnicity of individuals within the culture of rurality. A key consideration is that interventions and strategies may be more effectively developed and implemented at the level of race/ethnicity while taking into account the access and use of information among rural populations.

This descriptive, cross-sectional study adds understanding to health-seeking behaviors among African Americans, Caucasians, and Hispanics who live in rural areas within selected regions of the United States. As previously stated, the overall intent of the study was not to support that fact that differences exist between rural and urban populations because it is known that there are differences but to better understand the behaviors of rural Americans. There were some demographic differences among the sample that tended to mirror the general population as Hispanics were younger and African Americans older than Caucasian participants.

African Americans reported more visits to their health care provider despite the fact that most participants reported their health as good or very good. Reasons for this difference are unclear. Although it may also be related to the fact that African Americans were significantly older, all participants identified their health care provider as a source of health information. Perhaps one of the glaring findings from the research is that less than half the sample reported *ever* looking for health information, with African Americans being less likely to have looked for this information. This finding is consistent with that reported by Tu[11] who suggests an overall decline in consumer health-seeking behaviors. This fact not only underscores the importance of providers as a source of health information but may also suggest the need for more effective partnerships with health insurers, both private and government funded. In the current sample, Hispanics were less likely to have any insurance, which suggests that alternate ways such as health navigation or community outreach may also be needed to reach this population.

Findings raise the issue of active information seeking versus passive information. That is, although participants may not have sought health information, they may have been exposed to it via the forms of media that they used. For example, participants in this sample watch television an average of 3.59 hours per day. They may have viewed programming on cancer or other health-related issues within the context of their viewing but were not actively seeking this information. Moreover, close to 40% of participants used print media (books, magazine, pamphlets); this can also be a source of passive health information. Documenting access to and use of passive health information is somewhat difficult, especially as it relates to health care outcomes and/or targeted interventions.

Active seekers of health-related information among this sample most frequently used the Internet and their health care provider. However, Hispanics were less likely to get information from their provider, which may be related to the fact that they had fewer visits to the provider than others. These findings raise another issue on how participants receive information from their provider. Traditionally, this information has been imparted during an office visit or perhaps through follow-up from the nurse. Technology provides additional patient-provider communication opportunities. However, only 25% wanted their provider to send them information on their health by e-mail.

Access to the Internet alone may not translate into increased health-seeking behaviors. It is important to understand the devices that are used to access the Internet and what activities people participate in while in the online environment, as this may influence how much information is accessible and the speed of access, as well as provide insights into how to better tailor and target health-related content. Few participants reported having smartphones (less than 40%) or tablet devices (less than 20%) that would allow them to access information regardless of their location. This fact must be considered within the context of a health care system that often directs patients to a Web site or sends information by text or e-mail. Although these participants can access the information, the timeliness in which the information reaches them may be compromised.

Lastly, in applying the findings of this study, it should be remembered that the data come from a cross section of participants from 3 states and therefore generalizability may be limited. The fact that less than 50% of participants actively sought health-related information in the past year made the cell sizes small for questions that specifically asked how they obtained the information. Finally, the intent of this study was not to assess how information was used to support or lead to behavior change, which is a critical issue for public health.

IMPLICATIONS FOR NURSING

Nurses form the foundation for providing patient education regardless of their practice setting. Nursing education has appropriately made the shift from brick and mortar classrooms in isolation to embedding the use of technology (eg, online classes, electronic books); yet, patients continue to be discharged with typed, mass-produced discharge instructions and summaries. Findings from the current study support the fact that rural participants have access to the Internet. Now, the focus must shift to match how the patient accesses and uses the Internet with how health information is disseminated in the online environment. Although issues of security in the online environment cannot be overlooked, it may be helpful to ask patients if they would like to receive e-mail updates or text messages on general (nonpatient specific) health care topics. These types of messages could take on a variety of formats and be sent using automated systems. The goal in this type of intervention is not to replace or discount the personal patient-provider interaction but provide an alternative for those who are comfortable in the online environment. One way to do this is to include a phone number or the e-mail of a provider who can be contacted for additional questions or follow-up. Although studies clearly support that the use of print media has declined over time,[11] a large portion of the current sample used print, along with TV, as an information source. Therefore, there is a need to use a multiplatform approach to the delivery of health-related information instead of the online environment in isolation.

Findings clearly show that there are disparities within disparities, although this was not the aim of the study. Previous reports have shown differences in demographic predictors between rural and urban populations.[13,22] This study highlights that disparities exist within rural populations and these differences may have implications for the manner of dissemination of health-related information and the uptake of the information. Education has been identified as a critical predictor of health-seeking behaviors[11]; there were differences in levels of education based on race/ethnicity within the study sample. This fact highlights the need to target and tailor messages using multiple platforms and that information must be at the appropriate literacy and numeracy level.

To this end, more research is needed on effectively structuring Web sites that are easily navigated by persons with low levels of education or health literacy, regardless of their race/ethnicity or geography[23,24]; this is critical because information seekers who become frustrated as they seek information are more likely to stop or give up on the search.[11] Additional research is needed on how individuals evaluate Web sites to ensure that the information is credible. Although there are resources to help the public evaluate credibility, it is unclear if the public is aware of these resources. Consistent with previous studies,[25] participants in the current study, regardless of age and race/ethnicity, used social networking sites (eg, Facebook) but were not likely to use the site for health information, were not likely to read health-related pop-up information online, and were not likely to download apps. Although these findings are not new,[13,23] more research is needed to understand adoption of these types of resources to disseminate information (passive) and then determine if the individuals use or revisit the resources when they are actively seeking information.

Lastly, nurse-led research in the area of patient communication channels within the technological age is lacking. Nurses, regardless of practice, research, or educational setting, must become more involved in the development of online patient-centered materials. Nurses should partner with software, Web content experts, and Web designers to ensure that information is understandable, at an appropriate literacy and numeracy level, and can be easily accessed.

REFERENCES

1. Niederdeppe J, Hornik RC, Kelly BJ, et al. Examining the dimensions of cancer-related information seeking and scanning behavior. Health Commun 2007;22(2): 153–67.
2. Nielsen J. Digital divide: the three stages. 2006. Available at: http://www.useit. com/alertbox/digital-divide.html. Accessed January 17, 2015.

3. Kontos EZ, Emmons KM, Puleo E, et al. Communication inequalities and public health implications of adult social networking site use in the United States. J Health Commun 2010;15(S3):216–35.
4. Clayman ML, Manganello JA, Viswanath K, et al. Providing health messages to Hispanics/Latinos: Understanding the importance of language, trust in health information sources, and media use. J Health Commun 2010;3:252–63.
5. Viswanath K, McCloud R, Minsky S, et al. Internet use, browsing, and the urban poor: Implications for cancer control. J Natl Cancer Inst Monogr 2013;2013(47): 199–205.
6. Kratzke C, Wilson S, Vilchis H. Reaching rural women: Breast cancer prevention information seeking behaviors and interest in Internet, cell phone, and text use. J Community Health 2013;38(1):54–61.
7. Rooks RN, Wiltshire JC, Elder K, et al. Health information seeking and use outside of the medical encounter: is it associated with race and ethnicity? Soc Sci Med 2012;74(2):176–84.
8. Thompson VL, Cavazos-Rehg P, Tate KY, et al. Cancer information seeking among African Americans. J Cancer Educ 2008;23(2):92–101.
9. Rutten LJ, Squires L, Hesse B. Cancer-related information seeking: hints from the 2003 Health Information National Trends Survey (HINTS). J Health Commun 2006; 11(Supplement 1):147–56.
10. Laz TH, Berenson AB. Racial and ethnic disparities in Internet use for seeking health information among young women. J Health Commun 2013;18(2):250–60.
11. Tu HT. Surprising decline in consumers seeking health information. 2011. Available at: http://hschange.org/CONTENT/1260/1260.pdf. Accessed January 17, 2015.
12. Lustria ML, Smith SA, Hinnant CC. Exploring digital divides: An examination of eHealth technology use in health information seeking, communication and personal health information management in the USA. Health Informatics J 2011; 17(3):224–43.
13. Fox S. Rural e-patients face access challenges. 2012. Available at: http://www.pewinternet.org/2012/11/26/rural-e-patients-face-access-challenges/. Accessed January 17, 2015.
14. Marketing Systems Group. GENESYS sampling solutions. 2015. Available at: www.m-s-g.com/web/genesys/index.aspx. Accessed January 17, 2015.
15. National Cancer Institute. Health Information National Trends Survey. 2015. Available at: http://hints.cancer.gov/. Accessed January 17, 2015.
16. The Pew Charitable Trust. The Pew Research Center. 2015. Available at: http://www.pewtrusts.org/en. Accessed January 17, 2015.
17. Lyons K. Final report: exploring use of cancer communication and information channels among diverse groups within American Cancer Society divisions. Gainesville (FL): Independent Data Collection Center; 2013.
18. Creative Research Systems. Computer assisted telephone interviewing. 2015. Available at: http://www.surveysystem.com/interviewing-cati.htm. Accessed January 17, 2015.
19. Apple. Start something new. 2015. Available at: http://www.apple.com/start-something-new/. Accessed January 17, 2015.
20. Facebook. Connect with friends and the world around you with Facebook. 2015. Available at: https://www.facebook.com/. Accessed January 17, 2015.
21. Viswanath K, Ackerson LK. Race, ethnicity, language, social class, and health communication inequalities: a nationally representative cross-sectional study. PLoS One 2011;6(1):e14550.

22. Richardson A, Allen JA, Xiao H, et al. Effects of race/ethnicity and socioeconomic status on health information-seeking, confidence, and trust. J Health Care Poor Underserved 2012;23(4):1477–93.
23. Atkinson NL, Saperstein SL, Pleis J. Using the Internet for health-related activities: Findings from a national probability sample. J Med Internet Res 2009;11(1):e4.
24. Viswanath K, Kreuter MW. Health disparities, communication inequalities, and eHealth. Am J Prev Med 2007;32(5 Suppl):S131–3.
25. Chou WY, Hunt YM, Beckjord EB, et al. Social media use in the United States: implications for health communication. J Med Internet Res 2009;11(4):e48.

Impact of Age and Comorbidity on Cervical and Breast Cancer Literacy of African Americans, Latina, and Arab Women

CrossMark

Costellia H. Talley, PhD[a],*, Karen Patricia Williams, PhD[b]

KEYWORDS

- Cervical cancer • Breast cancer • Literacy • Age-adjusted comorbidity
- Chronic disease

KEY POINTS

- Cancer literacy and cancer screening rates are lower among medically underserved populations.
- Comorbidities (chronic medical conditions) may serve as a barrier to timely and appropriate cancer screening, particularly for African American women.
- Rates of screening are particularly low for foreign-born individuals who emigrated to the United States recently or who are less acculturated.
- Health literacy about breast and cervical cancer can improve screening, reduce burden, and improve health outcomes.
- Health care providers should consider age and comorbidity when designing screening interventions for underserved populations.

INTRODUCTION

Appropriate screening and early detection can significantly reduce breast and cervical cancer–associated morbidity and mortality, and the US Preventive Services Task Force,[1,2] American Cancer Society (ACS), American College of Obstetricians and

Disclosures: None.
This work was supported by the National Institutes of Health National Institute for Nursing Research (R01NR011323) and (R21NR010366).
[a] College of Nursing, Michigan State University, 1355 Bogue Street, Room C-247, East Lansing, MI 48824, USA; [b] Department of Obstetrics, Gynecology & Reproductive Biology, Michigan State University, 965 East Fee Road, Room A626, East Lansing, MI 48824, USA
* Corresponding author.
E-mail address: talleyc@msu.edu

Gynecologists, and several other national guidelines recommend regular screening.[3-5] This study uses the ACS guidelines for breast and cervical cancer screening, which are depicted in **Tables 1** and **2**. Many women do not obtain breast and cervical cancer screening at recommended regular intervals and experience delays in diagnostic follow-up after an abnormal mammogram.[6-9] Untimely screening and inappropriate follow-up after an abnormal mammogram increase the risk for late-stage diagnosis and larger-sized tumors.[8,9] Late-stage diagnosis negatively affects treatment, disease course, and survival.[10,11] Approximately 33% of eligible women (aged 40 years and older) have not received breast cancer screening within the past 2 years.[12] Breast cancer screening rates are lowest in women who are uninsured (38%), followed by immigrant women who have been in the United States for less than 10 years (39.9%). In 2013, 11% of women (aged 21–65) had not been screened for cervical cancer in the previous 3 years.[12,13] Cervical cancer screening has been consistently lower in women who are uninsured (61%), recent immigrants (66%), and women with education level less than high school (69%).

Several factors contribute to low breast and cervical cancer screening rates, including low socioeconomic status, low educational attainment, membership in a minority race/ethnic group, foreign-born or immigrant status, lack of a regular care provider, lack of a doctor's recommendation, lack of health care access, inconvenience, cultural beliefs, and lack of social support.[14,15] Lower screening rates in immigrant women may be partially attributed to language barriers (English proficiency). Limited English proficiency can lead to decreased access to health care, dissatisfaction with care, and decreased quality of care, and limit knowledge about cancer prevention and screening guidelines.[14-20] For example, in a study examining mammography screening among "Asian Indian" women, researchers reported that length of stay in

Table 1	
Comparison of US Preventive Services Task Force (USPSTF) and American Cancer Society (ACS) screening guidelines for breast cancer for women at average risk	
USPSTF	**ACS**
Biennial screening mammography beginning at age 50	Annual screening mammography beginning at age 40
Not enough evidence to support assessing the additional benefits of screening mammography in women past age 74	Annual screening mammography for as long as a woman is in good health
Recommends against health care providers teaching women how to perform breast self-examination	Breast self-examination is optional Beginning in their early 20s, women should be told about the benefits and limitations of breast self-examination. Instructions should be given by their health provider to women who choose to do breast self-examination
Evidence is insufficient for assessing the additional benefits of clinical breast examination beyond screening mammography in women 40 y or older	Recommends clinical breast examination every 3 y for women in their 20s and 30s, and annually for women aged 40 and older
Insufficient evidence to support the additional benefits and harms of MRI as a screening method for breast cancer	In addition to screening mammography, annual MRI screening is recommended for women with >20% lifetime risk of breast cancer

Data from Refs.[1,12,114]

Table 2
Comparison of USPSTF and ACS screening guidelines for cervical cancer for women at average risk

USPSTF	ACS
Cervical cancer screening should begin at age 21 y, regardless of the age of sexual initiation or other risk factors	Cervical cancer screening should begin at age 21 y, regardless of the age of sexual initiation or other risk factors
Screening recommended for women age 21–65 y with Pap test every 3 y or, for women age 30–65 y who want to lengthen the screening interval, screening with a combination of Pap test and HPV testing every 5 y	Screening recommendations by age group: Aged 21–29 y, screening with Pap test alone every 3 y, no testing for HPV unless abnormal Pap test; those aged 30–65 y should be screened with Pap test and HPV testing every 5 y (preferred) or Pap test alone every 3 y (acceptable)
Recommends against screening in women >65 y who have had adequate prior screening and are not otherwise at high risk for cervical cancer	Women >65 y who have had regular screenings with normal results should not be screened
Recommends against screening for cervical cancer in women who have had a hysterectomy with removal of the cervix and who do not have a history of a high-grade precancerous lesion or cervical cancer	Women who have had their uterus and cervix removed in a hysterectomy and have no history of cervical cancer or precancer should not be screened

Abbreviations: HPV, human papillomavirus; Pap, Papanicolaou.

Data from Moyer VA. Screening for cervical cancer: U.S. preventive services task force recommendation statement. Ann Int Med 2012;156(12):880–91; and American Cancer Society. New screening guidelines for cervical cancer. 2012. Available at: http://www.cancer.org/cancer/news/new-screening-guidelines-for-cervical-cancer. Accessed January 10, 2015.

the United States, marital status, knowledge of mammogram guidelines, age, having health insurance, physician recommendations, and number of relatives who had a mammogram were positively associated with having a mammogram within the past 2 years.[21] These findings suggest that women who have difficulty understanding spoken recommendations about breast and cervical cancer screening may be at risk for nonadherence to screening guidelines.[22] Knowledge (health literacy) about breast and cervical cancer and the benefits of screening are important determinants in screening adherence.[23,24]

Health literacy is a strong predictor of cancer screening rates. Health literacy is defined as a "wide range of skills and competencies that people develop to seek out, comprehend, evaluate, and use health information and concepts to make informed choices, reduce health risks, and increase quality of life."[25] Women with limited health literacy and limited English proficiency may have difficulty understanding screening guidelines and accessing and navigating the health care system, and difficulty with clinical decision making.[26] Moreover, because provider recommendation is an important factor in obtaining cancer screening, limited health literacy affects patient/provider communication. Low health literacy is associated with limited awareness about cancer screening, lack of desire for screening, and limited access to care.[27–29]

There is also evidence that comorbidities often serve as a barrier to timely and appropriate cancer screening.[30,31] Some studies document that specific comorbidities are an independent risk factor for cancer (eg, diabetes, hypertension).[32–34] For

Table 3 Age-adjusted Charlson comorbidity index scoring	
Score	**Comorbid Condition**
1	Myocardial infarction
	Congestive heart failure
	Cerebral vascular disease
	Peripheral vascular disease
	Dementia
	Chronic obstructive pulmonary disease
	Connective tissue disease
	Peptic ulcer disease
	Mild liver disease
2	Diabetes
	Hemiplegia
	Moderate/severe renal disease
	Diabetes with end-organ damage
	Any solid tumor
	Leukemia
	Lymphoma
3	Moderate/severe liver disease
6	Metastatic solid tumor
	AIDS
Age (y)	
41–50	1 point
51–60	2 points
61–70	3 points
≥71	4 points

example, women with diabetes are at increased risk for development of cancer and are 40% more likely to die from breast cancer than women who do not have diabetes.[35,36] In addition, women with diabetes are less likely to obtain breast and cervical cancer screening than women who do not have diabetes.[31,37] In one study, women with cardiovascular and lung disease were less likely to be up to date on breast cancer screening, and women with diabetes, arthritis, and hypertension were less likely to be up to date with cervical cancer screening when compared with women without comorbidities.[38]

Although there is evidence that regular breast and cervical cancer screening, and timely follow-up of abnormal tests, lead to decrease mortality,[39–42] racial/ethnic minority women, particularly immigrant women, continue to underuse cancer screening. Given the long-standing low screening rates of racial/ethnic minorities and the increasing number of immigrants to the United States, information that contributes to our understanding of factors that contribute to lower screening rates is important.[43–45] Moreover, information obtained from this study may be helpful in understanding screening patterns and facilitation of timely and appropriate screening. The present study addressed this need by examining the association between age, comorbid conditions, and breast and cervical cancer literacy of African American, Latina, and Arab women. These populations were selected for this study because they have lower screening rates, African American and Latina women have higher cancer-related mortality rates than white women, and Latina and Arab women are among the largest group of United States immigrants.[43] In addition, Michigan is among the states with the largest percentage increase of immigrants and has one of the largest concentrations of Arab Americans.[43,46,47] Few studies have addressed the association between age, comorbidity, and cancer health literacy in a sample of African American, Latina, and Arab women.

BREAST AND CERVICAL CANCER

For women in the United States, breast cancer is the most common cancer and the second leading cause of cancer death. In 2015, 231,840 new cases of invasive breast cancer are expected to be diagnosed and 40,290 women are expected to die of the disease.[48] Routine breast cancer screening can reduce morbidity and mortality from late-stage diagnosis and treatment.[49,50] Some women experience a delay in follow-up after an abnormal mammogram.[51]

Despite having a lower incidence of breast cancer than white women (**Fig. 1**), African American, Latina, and Arab women are more likely to be diagnosed at a younger age, more advanced stage of disease, and to have more aggressive forms of breast cancer.[52–56] Advanced stage of cancer diagnosis has been attributed to lower screening rates, inadequate knowledge about screening guidelines, and delayed follow-up for abnormal findings.[57,58] Studies have reported that racial/ethnic minority and low-income women are more likely to delay follow-up.[51,59–61] For example, in a study of African American, Latina, Asian, and white women, influential factors were reported to be African American ethnicity, income, perceived discrimination, not fully understanding the results of the mammogram, and being notified of abnormal findings by letter or phone instead of in-person.[61] A 3- to 6-month delay in treatment of breast cancer can reduce survival, and delays of longer than 1 year increase the odds of lymph node metastasis and larger tumors.[62,63] Breast cancer is the most commonly diagnosed cancer and the leading cause of cancer death in Latinas.[54] African American women are more likely to die of cancer than women of any other racial/ethnic group.[48] Arab American women have similar stage, age, and hormone receptor status as African Americans, but a better survival rate.[52,64]

In 2015, 12,900 new cases of invasive cervical cancer are expected to be diagnosed, and 1400 are expected to die of the disease.[48] More than half of cervical cancer deaths occur in women who have never been screened or women who have not been

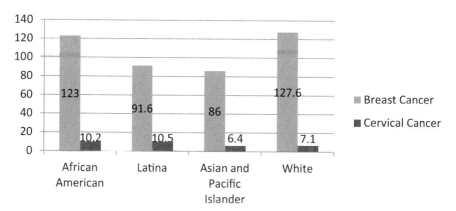

Fig. 1. Breast and cervical cancer incidence rates by race/ethnicity. Rates are per 100,000 population and age adjusted to the 2000 United States standard population. (*Data from* American Cancer Society. Incidence—North American Association of Central Cancer Registries, 2014. Mortality—US mortality data. 2015. Available at: http://www.cancer.org/research/cancerfactsstatistics/cancerfactsfigures2015/index. Accessed April 20, 2015.)

screened in the previous 5 years.[48] Cervical cancer is preventable with early detection and removal of precancerous cervical lesions.[48,65] Routine cervical cancer screening (Papanicolaou [Pap] test) or a human papillomavirus test allows for the detection of precancerous lesions that can be treated before progression to cancer. In addition, the time interval between cervical cancer screening, diagnosis, and treatment has a significant negative impact on health outcomes.[65] A longer interval between diagnostic identification of a precancerous lesion and treatment results in later-stage disease, decreased survival, and increased economic cost (to individual and society).[66,67] In women with a precancerous lesion who receive timely and appropriate evaluation, treatment, and follow-up, the probability of survival is almost 100%.[12] Racial ethnic minorities are less likely to meet the timeliness diagnostic interval.

The incidence of cervical cancer in the United States is highest in Latinas (10.5), followed by African American women (10.2) (see **Fig. 1**).[48,54,55] African American women are twice as likely as white women to die of cervical cancer (**Fig. 2**).[55] Available information in the literature about cervical cancer in Arab women indicates that in most Arab countries, cervical cancer is the second most common malignancy.[68] Studies examining cervical cancer among Arab American women indicate that cervical cancer screening is lower among Arab women than in the general population.[69] Studies also report that Arab women have a lower level of knowledge about cervical cancer.[70,71]

These findings suggest that early detection and treatment by adherence to established screening guidelines are critical to reducing morbidity and mortality in breast and cervical cancer. For example, women who receive cervical cancer screening within 3 to 36 months before cervical cancer diagnosis have a lower mortality rate.[39] However, many women do not adhere to these guidelines and many are not aware of them.[72,73] There is thus a clear need to identify factors that affect screening for women of racial/ethnic minority, particularly among immigrants and individuals with limited English proficiency, to improve cancer screening rates.

BREAST AND CERVICAL CANCER SCREENING, LITERACY, AGE, AND COMORBIDITY

Symptomatic presentation is often the most common route for a cancer diagnosis. Screening, testing an individual who has no symptoms,[12] allows for early detection

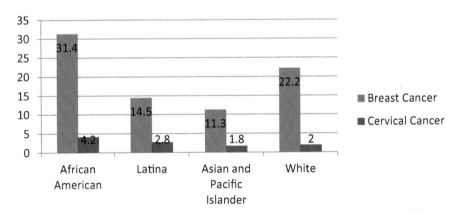

Fig. 2. Breast and cervical cancer mortality rates by race/ethnicity. Rates are per 100,000 population and age adjusted to the 2000 United States standard population. (*Data from* American Cancer Society. Incidence—North American Association of Central Cancer Registries, 2014. Mortality—US mortality data. 2015. Available at: http://www.cancer.org/research/cancerfactsstatistics/cancerfactsfigures2015/index. Accessed April 20, 2015.)

of disease. In 2013, 65.9% of United States women reported having a mammogram within the past 2 years.[12] Race/ethnicity and immigration status play a role in predicting breast and cervical cancer screening. Mammography rates are particularly low for foreign-born individuals who emigrated to the United States more recently or who are less acculturated (living in the United States <10 years) (39.9%) and uninsured women (38%).[12,74] The Pap test screening rate over the past 3 years for United States women is 80.1%. Similar to mammogram use, Pap test use was lowest in recent immigrants (65.9%) and uninsured women (60.6%).[12]

Knowledge (health literacy) about screening and its benefits is an important determinant of screening. One in 5 adults in the United States do not have the basic literacy skills to function sufficiently in our society, particularly in health care.[26] As health care consumers, these individuals often do not have the necessary information to make appropriate health care decisions. Underuse of breast and cervical cancer screening is associated with lower health literacy, particularly in ethnic/racial minorities. In a study examining the relationship between health literacy and screening mammography, health literacy had the strongest association with mammography screening.[75] Low health literacy contributes to social inequities and poor health outcomes,[76] and influences decision making about cancer screening and prevention.

In a study assessing cervical cancer screening in underserved African American women and Latinas, screening was low; Latina and older women were less likely to adhere to screening guidelines. Age, knowledge of screening recommendations, and having a regular health care provider were independently associated with both breast and cervical cancer screening in a sample of Latinas.[72] Similar results in this patient population have been reported by other researchers.[27,77–79] Knowledge about screening recommendations is also low in Arab women, and some studies indicate that even in women with adequate knowledge, screening is low.[57,68,80–83]

The risk of breast cancer increases with age. Aging is also associated with an increased risk of comorbidities and cancer. There are conflicting reports on the association between age, comorbidity, and cancer screening. Some studies report that comorbidity has little effect on the use of screening mammography and Pap testing, whereas others indicate that specific comorbidities increase the likelihood of timely cancer screening (eg, hypertension, digestive disorders).[38,84,85] These researchers suggest that individuals with comorbid conditions have more contact with the health care system and are more likely to be screened. Others suggest that women with comorbid conditions are less likely to be screened because of competing demands, and suggest that comorbid condition competes with the time and focus of the health care provider, and that it has an impact on the individual's resources. Diabetes has been consistently related to cancer screening rates.[86–88]

Low-income and African American women are more likely to have 2 or more comorbidities than white women. This study examined the association between age, comorbid conditions, and breast and cervical cancer literacy among medically underserved women (ie, African American, Latina, and Arab). To meet the needs of women with lower utilization of screening (racial/ethnic minorities, immigrants, low income) will require that clinicians understand the factors that contribute to lower screening rates.

METHODS
Design

This study used a quantitative, descriptive design. Breast and cervical cancer literacy, age, and comorbidity were evaluated to examine the association between age, comorbid conditions, and breast and cervical cancer literacy of African American, Latina, and Arab women.

Participants

This study used a purposive sample of women who participated in the community-based Kin Keeper[SM] Cancer Prevention Intervention studies, previously described in detail.[89–91] The studies were approved by the Michigan State University Institutional Review Board. Criteria for inclusion in the current study included: (1) female sex, (2) older than 40 years, and (3) self-identified as African American, Latina, or Arab. Inclusion criteria yielded a total sample of 371 women (African American = 161; Latina = 107; Arab = 103). For the original study, inclusion criteria were: female, age 21 to 70, self-identifies as African American, Latina, or Arab, receiving services from community health workers (CHWs) from 1 of the 3 community-based organizations, biological mother and grandmothers of the same race/ethnicity, willingness to recruit members of her female adult family to participate in a home education visit, and completion of 2 home-based educational sessions on breast and cervical cancer prevention and control.

Procedure

Participants were recruited from community-based organizations affiliated with the Detroit Department of Health and Wellness Promotion including: (1) Village Health Worker Program, (2) Community Health and Social Services, and (3) the Arab Community Center for Economic and Social Services. In brief, CHWs recruited women (age ≥21) of their respective race (African American, Latina, Arab) from their public health case load for 2 home-based educational sessions. After signing the consent form during first home visit, the CHW and family unit completed the Historical Background Questionnaire and the breast cancer assessment (baseline). After completion of a pretest to assess breast cancer literacy, the educational intervention was delivered, followed by a posttest. During the second educational session the second posttest was delivered, followed by the cervical educational session and a posttest. During the second visit, participants also completed a personal action plan.

Questionnaire Items

Sociodemographic characteristics
Demographic factors on marital status, income, education, employment status, and age were considered.

Comorbidities
Data about comorbidities were obtained by the participants' response to the question, "Have you ever been told by a doctor or health professional that you had?" Based on the comorbidities, all patients were assigned a comorbidity score based on the Age-adjusted Charlson Index score as described by Charlson and colleagues.[92,93] The overall score is a weighted summation of medical conditions and age, with higher scores indicating a higher medical comorbidity (**Table 3**).

Breast and cervical cancer literacy
Breast cancer literacy was assessed with the Breast Cancer Literacy Assessment Tool (Breast-CLAT), a 35-item assessment instrument that measures functional breast cancer literacy in 3 domains: (1) awareness (items 1–6), (2) knowledge and screening (items 7–19), and (3) prevention and control (items 20–35).[94] The Breast-CLAT uses a multiple choice and true/false format and is scored as a binary variable (0 = incorrect, 1 = correct). Scores range from 0 to 35, with higher scores indicating a higher level of

functional breast cancer literacy. The instrument has been validated in English, Spanish, and Arabic, with a total scale Cronbach $\alpha = .73$.[94] The total scale reliability was highest in African Americans and lowest in Latinas (.81 and .61, respectively).[94,95] Breast-CLAT total and subscale scores were assessed.

Cervical cancer literacy was assessed with the Cervical Cancer Literacy Assessment Tool (C-CLAT).[95,96] This 16-item instrument contains 3 domains: (1) Awareness, (2) Knowledge and Screening, and (3) Prevention and Control.[97] The items are scored as a binary variable (0 = incorrect, 1 = correct). Scores range from 0 to 16, with higher scores indicating better literacy. The internal consistency of the C-CLAT was high (0.72). The C-CLAT reliabilities in African American, Latina, and Arab women were 0.73, 0.76, and 0.60, respectively. The C-CLAT scores were assessed by subscale and total scores.

Data Analysis

Data were analyzed using Stata (version 12.1) software.[98] Descriptive statistics (mean, standard deviation [SD], frequency, and proportion as appropriate) were used to describe the sample, including sociodemographic characteristics and comorbidities by racial/ethnic group. Analysis of variance (ANOVA), multivariate analysis of variance (MANOVA), and Tukey Honestly Significant Difference (HSD) post hoc tests were conducted to evaluate the effect of age-adjusted comorbidity on breast and cervical cancer literacy, plus measure the combined effect of age-adjusted comorbidity and race on breast and cervical cancer literacy. The main factors of interest were age-adjusted comorbidity and race, both categorical variables. This analysis was used given the likelihood that the dependent variables (ie, breast and cervical cancer literacy) are related to one another. Also, a 2-way MANOVA allowed for not only tests of the main effects of the independent variables (ie, age-adjusted comorbidity and race) but also for possible interaction effects between these variables, which is important given the relatively high co-occurrence of low breast and cervical cancer literacy in these populations. The use of MANOVA also reduces the risk of type I errors, which are more common with the use of repeated ANOVA. The Box test of equality was used to test the assumption of homogeneity of variance-covariance matrices, and the Levene test of equality was used to test the assumption of equality of variances. No significant violations to these assumptions were noted. Statistical significance was based on the Wilks λ statistic, and partial η^2 statistics were reported to illustrate effect size. The Tukey HSD tests were used to test all pairwise comparisons. The statistical significance of each result was evaluated according to its P value ($P<.05$ being significant) (Polit and Beck, 2012).

RESULTS

The sample included 371 women ranging in age from 41 to 101 years. African American women were more likely to be unmarried (**Table 4**). Participants were also dichotomized into 3 groups based on age-adjusted comorbidity scores: (1) low = 0 to 1 (n = 153); (2) mild = 2 to 3 (n = 144); and (3) severe = greater than 3 (n = 74).[99] The 2 most common comorbidities were hypertension and diabetes.

The distribution of age-adjusted comorbidity, and breast and cervical cancer literacy scores (total and subscale scores) are summarized in **Table 5**. ANOVA was conducted to compare age-adjusted comorbidity and the breast and cervical cancer literacy scores. Results of the ANOVA for breast cancer literacy (Breast-CLAT total scores) indicated that literacy was significantly different between groups ($F(2,367) = 17.31$, $P<.01$). Similarly, age-adjusted comorbidity scores indicated that

Table 4
Sociodemographic characteristics and comorbidities by racial/ethnic group (N = 371)

Variables	African American (n = 161)	Latina (n = 107)	Arab American (n = 103)
Age, years (mean ± SD)	53 ± 9	51 ± 9	53 ± 11
Marital status			
Married, n (%)	42 (27)	69 (66)	80 (78)
Education, n (%)			
<High school, n (%)	14 (9)	79 (74)	43 (42)
High school/GED, n (%)	53 (33)	17 (16)	37 (36)
>High school	93 (58)	10 (9)	22 (21)
Income,[a] n (%)			
<$9999	28 (18)	62 (60)	43 (43)
$10,000–$19,999	38 (24)	20 (19)	32 (32)
$20,000–$39,999	49 (31)	18 (17)	15 (15)
≥$40,000	43 (27)	4 (4)	10 (10)
Employment status,[a] n (%)			
Employed	99 (61)	47 (45)	19 (19)
Unemployed	62 (39)	57 (55)	83 (81)
Age-adjusted Charlson Comorbidity Index (ACC), n (%)			
Low (ACC 0–1)	56 (35)	47 (44)	50 (49)
Mild (ACC 2–3)	70 (43)	44 (41)	30 (29)
Severe (ACC >3)	35 (22)	16 (15)	23 (22)
Total no. of comorbid conditions			
Median	2	2	2
Range	0–6	0–5	0–5

Abbreviations: GED, General Education Development certificate; SD, standard deviation.
[a] ≠ 100 because of missing data.

Table 5
Means and standard deviations of age-adjusted comorbidity, breast cancer literacy, and cervical cancer literacy by racial/ethnic group (N = 371)

Measure	Racial/Ethnic Group			Total Sample
	African American (n = 161)	Latina (n = 107)	Arab (n = 103)	
Age-adjusted comorbidity (Mean ± SD)	3 ± 2	2 ± 2	2 ± 2	2 ± 2
Breast Cancer Literacy (mean ± SD)				
Total score	22 ± 4.8	19 ± 4.3	22 ± 3.8	21 ± 4.6
Awareness	4 ± 1.0	4 ± 3	3 ± 1	4 ± 1
Prevention	10 ± 3	12 ± 4	12 ± 2	11 ± 2
Screening	7 ± 2	7 ± 2	8 ± 2	7 ± 2
Cervical Cancer Literacy (mean ± SD)				
Total score	10 ± 3	10 ± 2	10 ± 2	10 ± 3
Awareness	1 ± 1	2 ± 1	1 ± 1	1 ± 1
Prevention	6 ± 2	6 ± 2	6 ± 2	6 ± 2
Screening	3 ± 1	3 ± 2	3 ± 2	3 ± 2

Abbreviation: SD, Standard deviation.

there was a significant difference between groups ($F(2, 367) = 3.08$, $P<.05$). Given the statistical omnibus of the ANOVA F test, MANOVA and Tukey HSD tests were conducted to examine pairwise contrasts.[100] For breast cancer literacy (total score), Tukey post hoc comparisons indicated that Latina scores (mean = 19, standard error [SE] = .43) were significantly different from those of African American (mean = 22, SE = .34) and Arab (mean = 22, SE = .43) women. Age-adjusted comorbidity scores were significantly different for African American women (mean = 1.9, SE = 0.06) compared with Latina women (mean = 1.7, SE = 0.06). Subscale scores were only significant for breast cancer awareness. For breast cancer awareness, scores for Arab women (mean = 2, SE = 0.2) were significantly different from those of African American (mean = 4, SE = 0.1) and Latina women (mean = 4, SE = 0.2). Comparisons of cervical cancer literacy (total scores and subscale scores) were not significant.

Effect of Age-Adjusted Comorbidity and Race on Breast Cancer Literacy

A factorial ANOVA was conducted to determine whether breast cancer literacy differed based on age-adjusted comorbidity and race (African American, Latina, and Arab). The 2-way factor analysis showed no significant main effect for age-adjusted comorbidity ($F(2,12) = 0.65$, $P>.05$). There was a significant main effect for race ($F(2,214) = 11$, $P<.01$), indicating that breast cancer literacy was influenced by race. The interaction between age-adjusted comorbidity and race was also significant ($F(2,70) = 3$, $P<.01$), indicating that differences in breast cancer literacy and age-adjusted comorbidity depend on race.

DISCUSSION

The purpose of this study was to assess the association between age-adjusted co-morbidity, and breast and cervical and literacy for African American, Latina, and Arab women. In this study, medical comorbidity as measured by the validated Age-adjusted Charlson Comorbidity Index indicated that it had a significant effect on health literacy. Medical comorbidities had a greater impact on breast cancer literacy of African American women than of Latina or Arab women. There are a limited number of studies that have used the Age-adjusted Charlson Comorbidity Index to assess the relationship between age, comorbidity, and breast and cervical cancer in an ethnically diverse sample of women. Most studies used the Age-adjusted Charlson Comorbidity Index as a predictor of mortality, survival prediction, and cancer treatment options.[99,101,102]

Studies examining the relationship between comorbidities and screening report that comorbidities are associated with adherence to breast and cervical cancer screening guidelines and a later stage at cancer diagnosis.[38,103] Vaeth and colleagues[104] evaluated comorbid conditions in women newly diagnosed with breast cancer, and reported that women with 2 or more comorbid conditions were more likely to be diagnosed at an advanced stage of disease. Similar results were reported by Kiefe and colleagues,[103] who examined the role of chronic disease as a barrier to screening for breast and cervical cancer. The researchers reported that selected chronic diseases (eg, heart disease, gastrointestinal disorders) contribute to lower screening rates. Studies also report the underuse of cancer screening by women with diabetes.[105,106] These findings suggest that age and comorbid conditions may contribute to lower literacy levels in African American women and delay in obtaining a screening test. This aspect is particularly important for African Americans because they are more likely to have chronic diseases.[107] For example, African Americans have higher rates of stroke (31%) and heart disease (23%) than whites.[108]

The women in this study demonstrated a moderate to relatively low level of breast cancer literacy (African American and Arab: mean = 22, SD = 4; Latina: mean = 19, SD = 4) and cervical cancer literacy (mean 10, SD = 2 for all groups). Similar results were reported by Dumenci and colleagues,[109] who reported limited cancer health literacy. In their study, 44% of African Americans believed that exposing a tumor to air during surgery would cause the tumor to spread, and that 23% of African Americans believe that rather than taking a pill twice a day as prescribed, taking it 3 times a day will help them get better more rapidly. This inadequate knowledge can affect an individual's decision to seek screening. Research by Garbers and Chiasson[79] indicates that Spanish-speaking women with inadequate health literacy are 16.7 times less likely to obtain cervical cancer screening.

There are limitations to this study that should be acknowledged. First, our findings may not generalize to other states, as our data come from only Michigan. However, Michigan has one of the largest Arab populations outside of the Middle East. Second, although the Age-adjusted Charlson Index is a valid and reliable instrument,[110] it does not represent functional impairment, which could influence cancer screening, particularly in older adults.[111–113] Future studies should also include functional impairment.

SUMMARY

The results of this study support previous studies of racial/ethnic minorities and immigrant populations, indicating overall low breast and cervical literacy (awareness, screening, and prevention). The influence of comorbidity on the stage at diagnosis and screening varies. However, our study supports the link between age-adjusted comorbidity in breast cancer literacy for African American women. This finding may be related to the fact that African Americans have a greater number of comorbidities. Breast cancer screening among African American women may be better targeted by considering comorbidities in addition to race. Increased knowledge of breast and cervical cancer could potentially lead to decreased stage at diagnosis and decreased mortality rates. Strategies to increase cancer screening at the primary and secondary levels are essential to the reduction of advanced stage at cancer diagnosis. These strategies should include improving cancer literacy and assessing comorbid conditions that may delay screening in medically underserved and immigrant populations.

ACKNOWLEDGMENTS

The authors would like to thank their community partners at the Detroit Department of Health and Wellness Promotion, and the Arab Community Center for Economic and Social Services.

REFERENCES

1. U.S. Preventive Services Task Force. Screening for breast cancer: U.S. Preventive Services Task Force recommendation statement. Ann Intern Med 2009; 151(10):716–26.
2. U.S. Preventive Services Task Force. Screening for cervical cancer: U.S. Preventive Services Task Force recommendation statement. Ann Intern Med 2012;156(12):880–91.
3. American Cancer Society. Breast cancer prevention and early detection. 2014. Available at: http://www.cancer.org/cancer/breastcancer/moreinformation/breastcancerearlydetection/breast-cancer-early-detection-toc. Accessed January 10, 2015.

4. Saslow D, Solomon D, Lawson HW, et al. American Cancer Society, American Society for Colposcopy and Cervical Pathology, and American Society for Clinical Pathology screening guidelines for the prevention and early detection of cervical cancer. CA Cancer J Clin 2012;62(3):147–72.

5. American College of Obstetricians and Gynecologists (ACOG). Practice bulletin no. 131: screening for cervical cancer. Obstet Gynecol 2012;120(5):1222–38.

6. Gierisch JM, Earp JA, Brewer NT, et al. Longitudinal predictors of nonadherence to maintenance of mammography. Cancer Epidemiol Biomarkers Prev 2010; 19(4):1103–11.

7. Hahn KM, Bondy ML, Selvan M, et al. Factors associated with advanced disease stage at diagnosis in a population-based study of patients with newly diagnosed breast cancer. Am J Epidemiol 2007;166(9):1035–44.

8. Taplin SH, Ichikawa L, Buist DS, et al. Evaluating organized breast cancer screening implementation: the prevention of late-stage disease? Cancer Epidemiol Biomarkers Prev 2004;13(2):225–34.

9. Zapka J, Taplin SH, Price RA, et al. Factors in quality care–the case of follow-up to abnormal cancer screening tests—problems in the steps and interfaces of care. J Natl Cancer Inst Monogr 2010;2010(40):58–71.

10. Braithwaite D, Tammemagi CM, Moore DH, et al. Hypertension is an independent predictor of survival disparity between African-American and white breast cancer patients. Int J Cancer 2009;124(5):1213–9.

11. Louwman WJ, Janssen-Heijnen ML, Houterman S, et al. Less extensive treatment and inferior prognosis for breast cancer patient with comorbidity: a population-based study. Eur J Cancer 2005;41(5):779–85.

12. American Cancer Society. Cancer prevention and early detection: facts and figures, 2015–2016. Atlanta (GA): American Cancer Society; 2015.

13. Centers for Disease Control. Millions of US women are not getting screened for cervical cancer. 2014. Available at: http://www.cdc.gov/media/releases/2014/p1105-vs-cervical-cancer.html. Accessed January 13, 2015.

14. Shelton RC, Jandorf L, King S, et al. Cervical cancer screening among immigrant Hispanics: an analysis by country of origin. J Immigr Minor Health 2012; 14(4):715–20.

15. Shirazi M, Bloom J, Shirazi A, et al. Afghan immigrant women's knowledge and behaviors around breast cancer screening. Psychooncology 2013;22(8): 1705–17.

16. Chavez LR, McMullin JM, Mishra SI, et al. Beliefs matter: cultural beliefs and the use of cervical cancer-screening tests. Am Anthropol 2001;103(4):1114–29.

17. De Alba I, Sweningson JM, Chandy C, et al. Impact of English language proficiency on receipt of pap smears among Hispanics. J Gen Intern Med 2004;19(9):967–70.

18. Goel MS, Wee CC, McCarthy EP, et al. Racial and ethnic disparities in cancer screening: the importance of foreign birth as a barrier to care. J Gen Intern Med 2003;18(12):1028–35.

19. Breen N, Rao SR, Meissner HI. Immigration, health care access, and recent cancer tests among Mexican-Americans in California. J Immigr Minor Health 2010;12(4):433–44.

20. Seid M, Stevens GD, Varni JW. Parents' perceptions of pediatric primary care quality: effects of race/ethnicity, language, and access. Health Serv Res 2003; 38(4):1009–31.

21. Somanchi M, Juon HS, Rimal R. Predictors of screening mammography among Asian Indian American women: a cross-sectional study in the Baltimore-Washington metropolitan area. J Womens Health (Larchmt) 2010;19(3):433–41.

22. Mazor KM, Williams AE, Roblin DW, et al. Health literacy and pap testing in insured women. J Cancer Educ 2014;29(4):698–701.

23. Bener A, Honein G, Carter AO, et al. The determinants of breast cancer screening behavior: a focus group study of women in the United Arab Emirates. Oncol Nurs Forum 2002;29(9):E91–8.

24. Soskolne V, Marie S, Manor O. Beliefs, recommendations and intentions are important explanatory factors of mammography screening behavior among Muslim Arab women in Israel. Health Educ Res 2007;22(5):665–76.

25. Zarcadoolas C, Pleasant A, Greer DS. Understanding health literacy: an expanded model. Health Promot Int 2005;20(2):195–203.

26. Davis TC, Williams MV, Marin E, et al. Health literacy and cancer communication. CA Cancer J Clin 2002;52(3):134–49.

27. Pagán JA, Brown CJ, Asch DA, et al. Health literacy and breast cancer screening among Mexican American women in South Texas. J Cancer Educ 2012;27(1):132–7.

28. Lindau ST, Basu A, Leitsch SA. Health literacy as a predictor of follow-up after an abnormal pap smear: a prospective study. J Gen Intern Med 2006;21(8):829–34.

29. Lindau ST, Tomori C, Lyons T, et al. The association of health literacy with cervical cancer prevention knowledge and health behaviors in a multiethnic cohort of women. Am J Obstet Gynecol 2002;186(5):938–43.

30. Lipscombe LL, Hux JE, Booth GL. Reduced screening mammography among women with diabetes. Arch Intern Med 2005;165(18):20902095.

31. Jiménez-Garcia RP, Hernandez-Barrera VM, Carrasco-Garrido PP, et al. Prevalence and predictors of breast and cervical cancer screening among Spanish women with diabetes. Diabetes Care 2009;32(8):1470–2.

32. Larsson SC, Mantzoros CS, Wolk A. Diabetes mellitus and risk of breast cancer: a meta-analysis. Int J Cancer 2007;121(4):856–62.

33. Michels KB, Solomon CG, Hu FB, et al. Type 2 diabetes and subsequent incidence of breast cancer in the Nurses' Health Study. Diabetes Care 2003;26(6):1752–8.

34. Salinas-Martínez AM, Flores-Cortés LI, Cardona-Chavarría JM, et al. Prediabetes, diabetes, and risk of breast cancer: a case-control study. Arch Med Res 2014;45(5):432–8.

35. Barone BB, Yeh HC, Snyder CF, et al. Long-term all-cause mortality in cancer patients with preexisting diabetes mellitus: a systematic review and meta-analysis. JAMA 2008;300(23):2754–64.

36. Lipscombe LL, Goodwin PJ, Zinman B, et al. The impact of diabetes on survival following breast cancer. Breast Cancer Res Treat 2008;109(2):389–95.

37. Lipscombe L, Fischer H, Austin P, et al. The association between diabetes and breast cancer stage at diagnosis: a population-based study. Breast Cancer Res Treat 2015;150(3):613–20.

38. Liu BY, O'Malley J, Mori M, et al. The association of type and number of chronic diseases with breast, cervical, and colorectal cancer screening in rural primary care practices. J Am Board Fam Med 2014;27(5):669–81.

39. Vicus D, Sutradhar R, Lu Y, et al. The association between cervical cancer screening and mortality from cervical cancer: a population based case-control study. Gynecol Oncol 2014;133(2):167–71.

40. Waterhouse H. National cancer screening programmes: risks, benefits and concerns. Pract Nurse 2013;43(7):44–8.

41. Gemignani ML. Breast cancer screening: why, when, and how many? Clin Obstet Gynecol 2011;54(1):125–32.

42. Onitilo AA, Engel JM, Liang H, et al. Mammography utilization: patient characteristics and breast cancer stage at diagnosis. Am J Roentgenol 2013;201(5):1057–63.

43. Camarota SA, Zeigler K. U.S. Immigrant population record 41.3 million in 2013. Washington, DC: Center for Immigration Studies; 2014.

44. Zong J, Batalova J. Frequently requested statistics on immigrants and immigration in the United States. 2015. Available at: http://www.migrationpolicy.org/article/frequently-requested-statistics-immigrants-and-immigration-united-states. Accessed April 18, 2015.

45. Brown W, Consedine N, Magai C. Time spent in the United States and breast cancer screening behaviors among ethnically diverse immigrant women: evidence for acculturation? J Immigr Minor Health 2006;8(4):347–58.

46. Auclair G, Batalova J. Middle Eastern and North African immigrants in the United States. Washington, DC: The Migration Policy Institute; 2013.

47. Schwartz K, Fakhouri M, Bartoces M, et al. Mammography screening among Arab American women in metropolitan Detroit. J Immigr Minor Health 2008; 10(6):541–9.

48. American Cancer Society. Cancer facts & figures: 2015. Atlanta (GA): American Cancer Society; 2015.

49. Malmgren JA, Parikh J, Atwood MK, et al. Impact of mammography detection on the course of breast cancer in women aged 40–49 years. Radiology 2012; 262(3):797–806.

50. Helvie MA, Chang JT, Hendrick RE, et al. Reduction in late-stage breast cancer incidence in the mammography era: implications for overdiagnosis of invasive cancer. Cancer 2014;120(17):2649–56.

51. Press R, Carrasquillo O, Sciacca RR, et al. Racial/ethnic disparities in time to follow-up after an abnormal mammogram. J Womens Health (Larchmt) 2008; 17(6):923–30.

52. Hensley Alford S, Schwartz K, Soliman A, et al. Breast cancer characteristics at diagnosis and survival among Arab-American women compared to European- and African-American women. Breast Cancer Res Treat 2009;114(2):339–46.

53. Iqbal J, Ginsburg O, Rochon PA, et al. Differences in breast cancer stage at diagnosis and cancer-specific survival by race and ethnicity in the United States. JAMA 2015;313(2):165–73.

54. American Cancer Society. Cancer Facts & figures for Hispanics/Latinos: 2012–2014. Atlanta (GA): American Cancer Society; 2012.

55. American Cancer Society. Incidence—North American Association of Central Cancer Registries, 2014. Mortality—US mortality data. 2015. Available at: http://www.cancer.org/research/cancerfactsstatistics/cancerfactsfigures2015/index. Accessed April 20, 2015.

56. Jandorf L, Fatone A, Borker PV, et al. Creating alliances to improve cancer prevention and detection among urban medically underserved minority groups. The East Harlem partnership for cancer awareness. Cancer 2006;107(8 Suppl):2043–51.

57. Arshad S, Williams KP, Mabiso A, et al. Evaluating the knowledge of breast cancer screening and prevention among Arab-American Women in Michigan. J Cancer Educ 2011;26(1):135–8.

58. McLaughlin JM, Anderson RT, Ferketich AK, et al. Effect on survival of longer intervals between confirmed diagnosis and treatment initiation among low-income women with breast cancer. J Clin Oncol 2012;30(36):4493–500.

59. Jones BA, Dailey A, Calvocoressi L, et al. Inadequate follow-up of abnormal screening mammograms: findings from the race differences in screening

mammography process study (United States). Cancer Causes Control 2005; 16(7):809–21.

60. Wujcik D, Shyr Y, Li M, et al. Delay in diagnostic testing after abnormal mammography in low-income women. Oncol Nurs Forum 2009;36(6):709–15.

61. Pérez-Stable EJ, Afable-Munsuz A, Kaplan CP, et al. Factors influencing time to diagnosis after abnormal mammography in diverse women. J Womens Health (Larchmt) 2013;22(2):159–66.

62. Olivotto IA, Gomi A, Bancej C, et al. Influence of delay to diagnosis on prognostic indicators of screen-detected breast carcinoma. Cancer 2002;94(8): 2143–50.

63. Richards MA, Westcombe AM, Love SB, et al. Influence of delay on survival in patients with breast cancer: a systematic review. Lancet 1999;353(9159): 1119–26.

64. Chouchane L, Boussen H, Sastry KS. Breast cancer in Arab populations: molecular characteristics and disease management implications. Lancet Oncol 2013; 14(10):e417–24.

65. Benard VB, Howe W, Royalty J, et al. Timeliness of cervical cancer diagnosis and initiation of treatment in the national breast and cervical cancer early detection program. J Womens Health (Larchmt) 2012;21(7):776–82.

66. Ashing-Giwa KT, Tejero JS, Kim J, et al. Cervical cancer survivorship in a population based sample. Gynecol Oncol 2009;112(2):358–64.

67. Subramanian S, Trogdon J, Ekwueme DU, et al. Cost of cervical cancer treatment: implications for providing coverage to low-income women under the Medicaid expansion for cancer care. Womens Health Issues 2010;20(6):400–5.

68. Ghazal-Aswad S, Hassan T, Badrinath P, et al. Screening for cervical cancer—the experience of the United Arab Emirates. Hamdan Medical Journal 2013; 6(1):105–10.

69. Darwish-Yassine M, Wing D. Cancer epidemiology in Arab Americans and Arabs outside the Middle East. Ethn Dis 2005;15(1 Suppl 1):S1–5, 8.

70. Al-Omran H. Measurement of the knowledge, attitudes, and beliefs of Arab-American adults toward cancer screening and early detection: development of a survey instrument. Ethn Dis 2005;15(1 Suppl 1):S1–15, 16.

71. Shah SM, Ayash C, Pharaon NA, et al. Arab American immigrants in New York: health care and cancer knowledge, attitudes, and beliefs. J Immigr Minor Health 2008;10(5):429–36.

72. Martinez-Donate AP, Vera-Cala LM, Zhang X, et al. Prevalence and correlates of breast and cervical cancer screening among a Midwest community sample of low-acculturated Latinas. J Health Care Poor Underserved 2013;24(4): 1717–38.

73. Lawsin C, Erwin D, Bursac Z, et al. Heterogeneity in breast and cervical cancer screening practices among female Hispanic immigrants in the United States. J Immigr Minor Health 2011;13(5):834–41.

74. Jacobs EA, Karavolos K, Rathouz PJ, et al. Limited English proficiency and breast and cervical cancer screening in a multiethnic population. Am J Public Health 2005;95(8):1410–6.

75. Komenaka IK, Nodora JN, Hsu CH, et al. Association of health literacy with adherence to screening mammography guidelines. Obstet Gynecol 2015; 125(4):852–9.

76. Zarcadoolas C, Greer DS, Pleasant A. Advancing health literacy: a framework for understanding and action. San Francisco (CA): Wiley, John & Sons, Inc; 2006.

77. Molina Y, Hohl S, Ko L, et al. Understanding the patient-provider communication needs and experiences of Latina and non-Latina white women following an abnormal mammogram. J Cancer Educ 2014;29(4):781–9.
78. Armin J, Torres CH, Vivian J, et al. Breast self-examination beliefs and practices, ethnicity, and health literacy: implications for health education to reduce disparities. Health Educ J 2014;73(3):274–84.
79. Garbers S, Chiasson MA. Inadequate functional health literacy in Spanish as a barrier to cervical cancer screening among immigrant Latinas in New York city. Prev Chronic Dis 2004;1(4):A07.
80. Alkhasawneh IM, Akhu-Zaheya LM, Suleiman SM. Jordanian nurses' knowledge and practice of breast self-examination. J Adv Nurs 2009;65(2):412–6.
81. Bener A, El Ayoubi HR, Moore MA, et al. Do we need to maximise the breast cancer screening awareness? Experience with an endogamous society with high fertility. Asian Pac J Cancer Prev 2009;10(4):599–604.
82. Montazeri A, Vahdaninia M, Harirchi I, et al. Breast cancer in Iran: need for greater women awareness of warning signs and effective screening methods. Asia Pac Fam Med 2008;7(1):6.
83. Taha H, Halabi Y, Berggren V, et al. Educational intervention to improve breast health knowledge among women in Jordan. Asian Pac J Cancer Prev 2010; 11(5):1167–73.
84. Heflin MT, Oddone EZ, Pieper CF, et al. The effect of comorbid illness on receipt of cancer screening by older people. J Am Geriatr Soc 2002;50(10):1651–8.
85. Yasmeen S, Xing G, Morris C, et al. Comorbidities and mammography use interact to explain racial/ethnic disparities in breast cancer stage at diagnosis. Cancer 2011;117(14):3252–61.
86. Chan W, Yun L, Austin PC, et al. Impact of socio-economic status on breast cancer screening in women with diabetes: a population-based study. Diabet Med 2014;31(7):806–12.
87. Fleming ST, Love MM, Bennett K. Diabetes and cancer screening rates among Appalachian and non-Appalachian residents of Kentucky. J Am Board Fam Med 2011;24(6):682–92.
88. Martinez-Huedo MA, Lopez de Andres A, Hernandez-Barrera V, et al. Adherence to breast and cervical cancer screening in Spanish women with diabetes: associated factors and trend between 2006 and 2010. Diabetes Metab 2012; 38(2):142–8.
89. Williams KP, Mabiso A, Todem D, et al. Differences in knowledge of breast cancer screening among African American, Arab American, and Latina women. Prev Chronic Dis 2011;8(1):A20.
90. Williams KP, Roman L, Meghea CI, et al. Kin KeeperSM: design and baseline characteristics of a community-based randomized controlled trial promoting cancer screening in Black, Latina, and Arab women. Contemp Clin Trials 2013;34(2):312–9.
91. Williams KP, Mullan PB, Todem D. Moving from theory to practice: implementing the Kin Keeper cancer prevention model. Health Educ Res 2009;24(2):343–56.
92. Charlson ME, Pompei P, Ales KL, et al. A new method of classifying prognostic comorbidity in longitudinal studies: development and validation. J Chronic Dis 1987;40(5):373–83.
93. Charlson M, Szatrowski TP, Peterson J, et al. Validation of a combined comorbidity index. J Clin Epidemiol 1994;47(11):1245–51.
94. Williams KP, Templin TN, Hines RD. Answering the call: a tool that measures functional breast cancer literacy. J Health Commun 2013;18(11):1310–25.

95. Rivera-Vasquez O, Mabiso A, Hammad A, et al. A community-based approach to translating and testing cancer literacy assessment tools. J Cancer Educ 2009;24(4):319–25.
96. Williams KP, Templin TN. Bringing the real world to psychometric evaluation of cervical cancer literacy assessments with Black, Latina, and Arab women in real-world settings. J Cancer Educ 2013;28(4):738–43.
97. Williams KP, Reckase M, Rivera-Vasquez O. Toward the development of cancer literacy assessment tools. Michigan J of Public Health 2008;2(1):21–31.
98. Stata. Stata data analysis and statistical software [computer program]. College Station (TX): StataCorp LP; 2013. Available at: http://www.stata.com/.
99. Robbins JR, Gayar OH, Zaki M, et al. Impact of age-adjusted Charlson comorbidity score on outcomes for patients with early-stage endometrial cancer. Gynecol Oncol 2013;131(3):593–7.
100. Lomax RG, Hahs-Vaughn DL. An introduction to statistical concepts. Third edition. New York: Taylor & Francis Group, LLC; 2012.
101. Koppie TM, Serio AM, Vickers AJ, et al. Age-adjusted Charlson comorbidity score is associated with treatment decisions and clinical outcomes for patients undergoing radical cystectomy for bladder cancer. Cancer 2008;112(11):2384–92.
102. Ouellette JR, Small DG, Termuhlen PM. Evaluation of Charlson-Age Comorbidity Index as predictor of morbidity and mortality in patients with colorectal carcinoma. J Gastrointest Surg 2004;8(8):1061–7.
103. Kiefe CI, Funkhouser E, Fouad MN, et al. Chronic disease as a barrier to breast and cervical cancer screening. J Gen Intern Med 1998;13(6):357–65.
104. Vaeth PA, Satariano WA, Ragland DR. Limiting comorbid conditions and breast cancer stage at diagnosis. J Gerontol A Biol Sci Med Sci 2000;55(10):M593–600.
105. Beckman TJ, Cuddihy RM, Scheitel SM, et al. Screening mammogram utilization in women with diabetes. Diabetes Care 2001;24(12):2049–53.
106. McBean AM, Yu X. The underuse of screening services among elderly women with diabetes. Diabetes Care 2007;30(6):1466–72.
107. Zonderman AB, Ejiogu N, Norbeck J, et al. The influence of health disparities on targeting cancer prevention efforts. Am J Prev Med 2014;46(3, Supplement 1):S87–97.
108. Kung HC, Hoyert DL, Xu JQ, et al. Deaths: final data for 2005. Natl Vital Stat Rep 2008;56(10):1–120. Available at: http://www.cdc.gov/nchs/data/nvsr/nvsr56/nvsr56_10.pdf.
109. Dumenci L, Matsuyama R, Riddle DL, et al. Measurement of cancer health literacy and identification of patients with limited cancer health literacy. J Health Commun 2014;19(Suppl 2):205–24.
110. de Groot V, Beckerman H, Lankhorst GJ, et al. How to measure comorbidity. a critical review of available methods. J Clin Epidemiol 2003;56(3):221–9.
111. Extermann M, Overcash J, Lyman GH, et al. Comorbidity and functional status are independent in older cancer patients. J Clin Oncol 1998;16(4):1582–7.
112. Wedding U, Rohrig B, Klippstein A, et al. Age, severe comorbidity and functional impairment independently contribute to poor survival in cancer patients. J Cancer Res Clin Oncol 2007;133(12):945–50.
113. Wu CC, Hsu TW, Chang CM, et al. Age-adjusted Charlson comorbidity index scores as predictor of survival in colorectal cancer patients who underwent surgical resection and chemoradiation. Medicine 2015;94(2):e431.

114. American Cancer Society. Breast cancer prevention and early detection. 2003. Available at: http://www.cancer.org/cancer/breastcancer/moreinformation/breastcancerearlydetection/breast-cancer-early-detection-toc. Accessed January 10, 2015.

Interactive Multimedia Tailored to Improve Diabetes Self-Management

Felecia G. Wood, PhD, RN, CNL[a],*, Elizabeth Alley[b], Spencer Baer[b], Rebecca Johnson, MLIS[c]

KEYWORDS

- Type 2 diabetes • Technology • Rural adults • Self-management • Health literacy
- Mobile applications

KEY POINTS

- Self-management of type 2 diabetes requires continuous complex decision making.
- Many rural dwellers struggle with health literacy.
- Mobile technology applications (apps) can offer ready access to health information.

Nearly 10% of the United States population has diabetes, and of these 29.1 million people with diabetes only 21 million have been diagnosed.[1] Most adults have been diagnosed with type 2 diabetes. Economically the impact of diabetes continues to soar, with 2012 data indicating combined direct and indirect costs of $245 billion.[1] Human costs associated with this chronic health problem are also devastating. Complications associated with diabetes can include blindness, amputation, painful neuropathy, and chronic kidney disease.

Diabetes, like many chronic illnesses, is more prevalent in rural than in urban areas.[2] Health disparities common in rural areas such as fewer health care providers,[2,3] lack of

Financial Support Disclosure: The technology used in this research was developed with financial support from the Walker Area Community Foundation (Walker County, AL), the Health Action Partnership of Walker County (Walker County, AL), and The University of Alabama (GR 23881) Capstone College of Nursing (Tuscaloosa, AL). Undergraduate students from The University of Alabama Computer-Based Honors Program contributed technical expertise in app development. Technical equipment was provided by The University of Alabama College of Arts & Sciences (Tuscaloosa, AL).
[a] The University of Alabama Capstone College of Nursing, Box 870358, Tuscaloosa, AL 35487-0358, USA; [b] The University of Alabama, Tuscaloosa, AL, USA; [c] Rochester Institute of Technology, Rochester, NY, USA
* Corresponding author.
E-mail address: fwood@ua.edu

transportation,[3] lower health literacy, and lower income[3] increase the challenges for effective self-management of diabetes. Navigating the daily requirements of life with diabetes requires much time, knowledge, a commitment to a healthy lifestyle, and an encouraging, accessible health care provider who facilitates the development of problem-solving skills. Individuals living with diabetes must make decisions regarding food intake, physical activity, medications, and health maintenance that are often based on brief initial education and infrequent visits to the health care provider, placing most of the responsibility for daily decisions regarding health on those living with diabetes.

Self-management education is necessary for those who hear the words "you have diabetes." Visions of relatives who experienced negative outcomes, frustration with a change in diet, and multiple daily injections may conjure up feelings of denial, anger, and depression as part of the fear of the unknown. For those who lack access to diabetes education, such as many rural dwellers, the fear continues. Even those who do participate in self-management education following the initial diagnosis struggle to maintain the momentum of daily vigilance over the long term. Consequently, most adults living with diabetes rely on quarterly visits to a health care provider who may not be adept at facilitating development of problem-solving skills, and who is rarely available to answer all self-management questions. Education handouts designed to teach skills for living with diabetes may not be easily understood, and may lead to further anxiety and confusion. For those living in rural areas, these challenges are magnified and contribute to a life expectancy reduced by 2 years for rural populations in comparison with urban dwellers.[4] Surprisingly, responses to the 2007 Behavioral Risk Factor Surveillance Survey indicated that rural dwellers exhibited better diabetes self-care behaviors than urban residents, even with the lack of resources typically available to those living in rural areas.[5]

Technology offers opportunities to increase knowledge and learn new skills. Most adults (85%) report owning a cell phone, and many of these individuals download and use applications[6] or seek health information online, particularly those living with chronic illnesses such as diabetes.[7] Although many mobile applications (apps) designed for people living with diabetes aim to enhance understanding of the disease, most are focused on blood glucose monitoring and recording; we were unable to locate any apps that provided a comprehensive, plain-language approach to self-management for those who live with type 2 diabetes and their loved ones. Mobile sources of reliable, evidence-based health information can bridge the gap between infrequent appointments with the health care provider.[8]

PURPOSE

A lack of available health care providers trained to help manage diabetes in rural areas, combined with patients who have not been taught about healthy living and have few available opportunities for additional health education, means that those living with diabetes are much more likely to have negative diabetes-related experiences. Given the challenges facing all adults living with diabetes, and the additional barriers faced by those living in rural areas who potentially also struggle with health literacy, a need exists for evidence-based accessible information. The purpose of this project was to pilot a program to improve self-management of type 2 diabetes in rural adults. Specifically, the project aims were to demonstrate that participants can effectively use the novel iOS-based, tailored intervention to improve diabetes self-management in a rural Southern US county, and to determine predictors of successful usage among this rural population living with type 2 diabetes.

TEAM APPROACH

The university from which the project originated included a team of faculty, staff, and undergraduate students. A College of Nursing faculty member engaged in research related to type 2 diabetes collaborated with a technical expert from the College of Arts and Sciences. The university offers a Computer-Based Honors Program (CBHP) for outstanding undergraduate students interested in expanding their technology knowledge and skill. These students are required to work with a faculty and/or staff person on a project for a semester. Two students were selected for this project, and both continued with the project for multiple semesters. Prior CBHP students had facilitated the evolution of this project from homemade videos and initial app development to app refinement and data collection and analysis. Multiple presentations and a published article describing strategies for selecting the best type of app for chronic disease self-management[8] have transpired from these collaborative activities over a period of 8 years. The staff and students gained experience with research and learned about diabetes self-management; the nurse faculty member described important components of diabetes self-management, and benefited from the technical expertise of the staff and students as they developed the app.

TECHNOLOGY

The content of an app can be native to, or reside within, the app; it may be provided from a Web site when the app is opened (eg, a news or weather app); or it may be hybrid, depending on some combination of the two. Given that those living in rural areas may not have reliable access to the Internet, a native application was selected for development. A native app does require Internet access for the initial download, but this can be accomplished using public Wi-Fi if the user does not have other access to the Internet. Once the app is downloaded, it maintains all functionality without connecting to the Internet.[8] Native apps can incorporate Web-based features, if desired, but for the purposes of this project a strictly native application was created. A native app is developed for a specific hardware manufacturer's device and is controlled by the manufacturer of that device; this app was developed for iOS devices such as the iPod Touch, iPad, and iPhone.

COMPONENTS OF THE APP

This evidence-based mobile application focused on basic diabetes self-management skills. All content was based on the 2012 Standards of Medical Care in Diabetes,[9] reflecting the most current evidence-based information available during the app development process. The developers worked to ensure that persons interacting with the app could identify with the people and activities featured in the application. For example, gender and ethnicity, language, and dress of the actors, in addition to the sites for video production, were carefully selected to reflect the lifestyle of rural dwellers.

The product of this faculty-staff-student collaboration was the native app *Diabetes 101*, developed for iOS devices including the iPod Touch, iPad, and iPhone using the XCode 5 with the iOS 7 SDK in Objective-C. Creation of a native app was particularly important for the intended audience (rural dwellers), as their access to Web-based technology may be unreliable, if available at all. All aspects of the app could be used multiple times to enable repetition of the important concepts for the person living with diabetes, and also permit family members and significant others to interact with the app repeatedly.

The app included 5 professionally developed videos depicting important self-management activities for persons living with type 2 diabetes. The videos addressed grocery store shopping, cooking, meeting with the health care provider, physical activity, and the emotional aspects of living with diabetes (**Fig. 1**). Each of the videos was preceded by a brief quiz to assess participant knowledge about the topic; if the question was answered incorrectly, the participant was immediately taken to the relevant video. If the question was answered correctly, participants had the option of viewing the video (**Fig. 2**). Each time the app was opened, pop-up reminders focused on typical diabetes self-management activities, such as "Have you checked your blood sugar today?" and "Have you made an appointment for a dilated eye examination?"

As health literacy is a concern for people living with chronic illness, participants also had access to a diabetes dictionary (**Fig. 3**) that included 50 common terms often used by health care providers when discussing type 2 diabetes, but defined in lay terms. Each term in the diabetes dictionary was accompanied by an audio recording of that word's pronunciation to enhance comprehension. Those with vision impairments also benefit from the audio definition. Participants were encouraged to engage in physical activity, and a brief self-assessment was provided to ensure they were healthy enough to increase physical activity; accompanying the self-assessment was a recommendation that the participant have a discussion with the health care provider regarding physical activity (**Fig. 4**).

METHODS

Diabetes 101 was beta-tested with 7 adults receiving care at a free clinic in a rural county in the southern United States. This county ranks next to last in health status indicators.[10] Of all residents of the state, 11.1% have diabetes. In the county in this study, 15% of residents had been diagnosed with diabetes.[11]

The research was approved by the university Institutional Review Board and by the director of the clinic where data were collected. Following written informed consent, participants were asked to complete data-collection tools assessing general health literacy (REALM[12] [Rapid Estimate of Adult Literacy in Medicine], a 66-item assessment completed by asking participants to read each word aloud), self-care activities (Summary of Diabetes Self-Care Activities,[13] a brief questionnaire assessing 5 aspects of diabetes self-management), self-efficacy (Diabetes Self-Efficacy,[14] an 8-item tool measuring confidence in performing activities necessary for diabetes self-management), diabetes knowledge (Diabetes Knowledge Test,[15] a 23-item assessment of general knowledge about diabetes), and a demographic questionnaire developed by the investigators.

Once data-collection tools were completed, participants were introduced to the iPod Touch technology and the *Diabetes 101* app. Education was provided to ensure that participants were comfortable using the technology and the app, and understood that Internet access was not required to use the app. Participants were asked to take the iPod Touch home for 2 weeks, use the technology as frequently as desired, and return to the clinic for post-tests, at which time all data-collection tools were repeated with the exception of demographic data. Participants were also asked to evaluate the technology following the 2-week data-collection period.

FINDINGS

Seven participants completed the 2-week intervention using the iPod Touch and all data-collection instruments. Fourteen individuals were approached for participation in the pilot project; 3 declined participation. Eleven individuals consented to

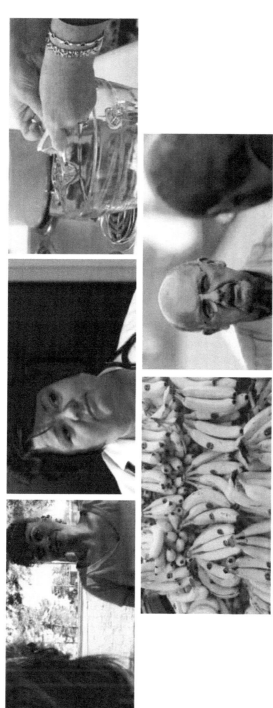

Fig. 1. Video topics.

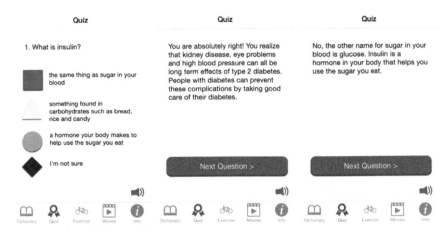

Fig. 2. Sample quiz item with responses.

participate in the research, but only 7 completed the intervention using the iPod Touch and data-collection instruments. As this was a pilot study, the sample size of 7 was deemed sufficient for the purposes of this initial research.

All participants had at least 11 years of formal education; ages ranged from 43 to 64 with a mean age of 50.1 years; 6 of the participants were Caucasian (83%) and 1 was African American (17%). Years since diagnosis with type 2 diabetes ranged from 1 to 24, with a mean of 14.1 years. Few participants were initially familiar with apps and i-Pod Touch technology.

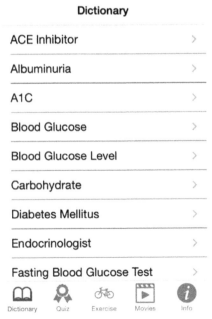
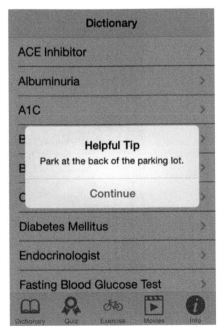
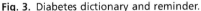

Fig. 3. Diabetes dictionary and reminder.

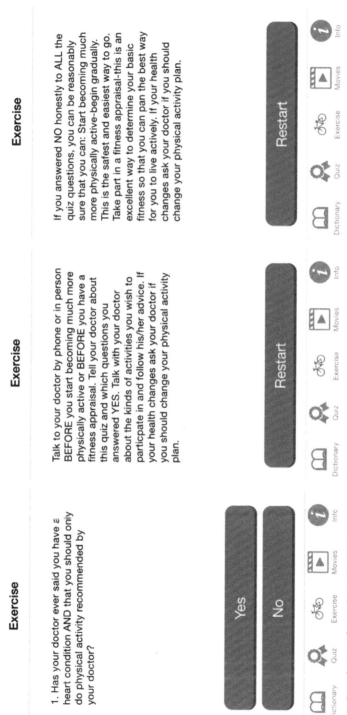

Fig. 4. Sample item from physical activity assessment.

Exercise

1. Has your doctor ever said you have a heart condition AND that you should only do physical activity recommended by your doctor?

Yes

No

Exercise

Talk to your doctor by phone or in person BEFORE you start becoming much more physically active or BEFORE you have a fitness appraisal. Tell your doctor about this quiz and which questions you answered YES. Talk with your doctor about the kinds of activities you wish to particpate in and follow his/her advice. If your health changes ask your doctor if you should change your physical activity plan.

Restart

Exercise

If you answered NO honestly to ALL the quiz questions, you can be reasonably sure that you can: Start becoming much more physically active–begin gradually. This is the safest and easiest way to go. Take part in a fitness appraisal–this is an excellent way to determine your basic fitness so that you can pan the best way for you to live actively. If your health changes ask your doctor if you should change your physical activity plan.

Restart

Dictionary   Quiz   Exercise   Movies   Info

Summary of Diabetes Self-Care Activities

Participants improved their self-care in some categories and decreased self-care activities in other categories (**Table 1**). For example, participants created a healthy eating plan, on average, 3.7 days per week before use of the app, which increased to 5.3 days per week following use of the app. Eating 5 fruits and vegetables daily decreased from an average of 4.1 days to 2.6 days per week. Engaging in 30 minutes of continuous physical activity only occurred 1.6 days per week for participants, and decreased slightly to 1.4 days following the intervention; the number of participants who took part in physical activity decreased from 4 to 2 during the data-collection period. All participants checked their blood sugar, but did not consistently check it as frequently as recommended by the health care provider (5.4 days prior; 5.7 days post). Two participants did not check their feet any days of the week pre- or postintervention; the remaining 5 participants checked their feet an average of 5.6 days before using the app and 5.2 days afterward. Before using the app, 5 participants never looked inside their shoes before putting them on; this improved to 4 participants after the intervention.

Rapid Estimate of Adult Literacy in Medicine

The REALM health literacy assessment asks participants to read 66 health-related terms. Correct pronunciation is assessed. All participants had clinically significant improvements following the intervention. The average REALM score preintervention was 45; following use of the app, the score was 65.5 of 66 items.

Diabetes Knowledge Test

Scores on the Diabetes Knowledge Test increased slightly following the intervention from 15.5 to 16.5 on the 23-item assessment of basic knowledge related to diabetes management.

Diabetes Self-Efficacy Scale

Participants were asked to rate how confident they were, on a scale of 1 to 10, at performing activities necessary for diabetes self-management. The self-efficacy, or confidence, was not a reflection of actually performing the activity, but an expression of confidence in the ability to perform the activity. Total average self-efficacy increased from 6.7 to 8.1 following the intervention. Participants expressed increased confidence in their ability to select appropriate foods to eat when they were hungry (from

Table 1 Summary of diabetes self-care activities (SDSCA)		
Tasks	Predeployment Days per Week	Postdeployment Days per Week
Healthful eating plan	3.7	5.3
5+ servings of fruits and vegetables	4.1	2.5
High-fat diet	2.5	2
30 minutes continuous exercise	1.6	1.4
Specific exercise session	2.1	1.3
Blood sugar testing	5.6	6.4
Check feet	4	3.25
Inspect inside of shoes	1.75	2.71

7.7 to 8.28). Confidence in exercising 15 to 30 minutes at least 4 to 5 times weekly increased from 4.7 to 5.57 following the intervention. Self-confidence in controlling diabetes, such that it does not interfere with what the participant wishes to do, increased from 6.57 to 7.43 following the intervention (**Fig. 5**).

Use of the App

Participants indicated comfort using the app, and enjoyed the flexibility of using it at any time in any location without needing Internet access. The ability to review the app multiple times was also viewed as a strength. All participants opened the app at least twice during the 2-week period, and some opened it as many as 16 times. Several participants expressed concern that they could not hear all of the dialogue in the videos. This drawback was corrected within the app following the intervention. Users particularly appreciated the videos, which showed "real people" experiencing the challenges of living with type 2 diabetes in a community environment at such sites as a grocery store, kitchen, walking trail, and the office of a health care provider.

DISCUSSION

This project demonstrated the feasibility of providing general diabetes self-management education using an interactive app technology that did not require Internet access. The use of videos is a beneficial strategy for demonstrating how to ask questions of the health care provider, shop for groceries and prepare food, engage in physical activity, and deal with the emotional challenges of diabetes.

Communication with health care providers during an office visit is not always effective. A discussion rarely occurs; instead, many patients wait for the health care provider to "prescribe" behaviors and medications. The videos in this mobile app

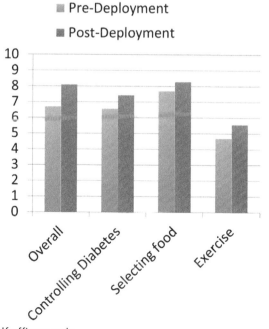

Fig. 5. Diabetes self-efficacy scale.

demonstrated a true conversation whereby the person seeking care comes prepared with questions and helps to guide the interaction.

The participants in this research had lived with diabetes an average of 14.1 years, yet clearly benefited from the self-management education included in this mobile app. Persons living with chronic health problems and their loved ones can benefit from readily accessible, mobile visual guides that demonstrate successful self-management strategies using a vocabulary that limits the use of medical terminology, portrayed by characters reflective of rural dwellers.

The 2-week time period during which the pilot project occurred for these participants likely was not sufficient to initiate and maintain changes in behaviors, but did lead to some change in many critical diabetes self-management activities.

These middle-aged rural dwellers had lived with type 2 diabetes for many years, on average, yet were not consistently performing many necessary self-management activities such as checking their feet, eating 5 fruits and vegetables daily, and monitoring blood sugar as recommended by their health care providers. Engagement in physical activity was minimal for these participants. The participants increased their knowledge about diabetes during the 2 weeks of app usage. Confidence in performing many diabetes self-management activities increased following use of the app, specifically in selecting appropriate foods, engaging in physical activity, and ensuring that diabetes self-management activities did not prevent the individual from enjoying desired activities, all of which are critical to effective self-management.

Participants enjoyed the interactive format of the quizzes, videos, and diabetes dictionary. Inclusion of "real people" who "looked like them" in the videos helped them to recognize that effective self-management is possible. Though somewhat frightening initially, the technology was not reported as an impediment to use of the app, which helped individuals living with type 2 diabetes and their loved ones to repeatedly review critical self-management strategies for a successful life change.

The small sample size in this study clearly limits the generalizability of the findings; replication with a larger sample is warranted. Geographic variation in data collection and similar testing among adults who are not rural dwellers will also be invaluable.

THE BIG PICTURE

For those living with diabetes or other chronic health problems, particularly those who live in rural areas or are medically underserved in other ways, knowledge that is applicable to daily life is critical for effective self-management. Success with self-management is unlikely when a person is handed printed reams of paper when exiting a health care provider's office with instructions to read and follow.

Learning and using health care terminology can be likened to learning a new language. Those who struggle with literacy likely also struggle with health literacy and understanding of the requisite knowledge and skills for managing a chronic illness. The necessary information and life skills may take time to assimilate, and a "one-and-done" education may be inadequate. Visual and auditory supplementation of the printed word will enhance success, as will the opportunity to engage in repetition of these learning sessions. Purchasing services to supplement the printed word may not be an option for those who lack insurance coverage for health education. Taking time away from work to devote time (and lost income) to self-management skills may be seen as unnecessary. Transportation may also be problematic if education services are not available locally.

Use of technology that is already available to most people in the form of smart-phones provides ready access, typically costs little to secure, and can be used at any time of day by multiple persons. Inclusion of dictionaries with written and spoken definitions of relevant terms may increase confidence in communicating with health care providers. Brief, "how-to" videos can also boost self-efficacy in the person living with a chronic illness and facilitate self-efficacy in their loved ones. Assessments of knowledge help validate understanding, and reminders for daily activities serve as prompts.

Accuracy of information included in any technology application must be assured by incorporating current evidence-based practice recommendations and clinical guidelines. Many resources are available on the Internet, but not all are current nor evidence-based, and most consumers who are looking for basic self-management assistance lack the ability to critically evaluate the quality of such resources.

How can the health care community contribute to improving outcomes for the millions of people who live with chronic illness each day? Equipping them with the knowledge, skills, and abilities to traverse the daily challenges of mundane, yet life-preserving activities—grocery shopping and cooking, conversing with a health care provider, initiating and maintaining a realistic physical activity plan, and dealing with the emotional highs and lows related to life with a chronic illness—can build confidence leading to success. Moreover, putting evidence-based resources, literally, in the palms of the hands of those in need may create the greatest impact on clinical practice. Mobile applications are not easily created, but resources exist in the health care and education communities to replace our outdated strategies for promoting healthy living in those with chronic illness.

REFERENCES

1. Centers for Disease Control and Prevention. National diabetes statistics report: estimates of diabetes and its burden in the United States, 2014. Atlanta (GA): U.S. Department of Health and Human Services; 2014.
2. Office of Rural Health Policy. Rural health facts. Available at: http://www.hrsa.gov/about/organization/bureaus/orhp. Accessed December 8, 2014.
3. National Rural Health Association. What's different about rural health care? Available at: http://www.ruralhealthweb.org/go/left/about-rural-health/what-s-different-about-rural-health-care. Accessed December 8, 2014.
4. Singh GK, Siahpush M. Widening rural-urban disparities in life expectancy, U.S., 1969-2009. Am J Prev Med 2014;46:e19–29.
5. Strom JL, Lynch CP, Egede L. Rural/urban variations in diabetes self care and quality of care in a national sample of US adults with diabetes. Diabetes Educ 2011;37:254–62.
6. Duggan M, Rainie L. Cell phone activities 2012. Available at: http://pewinternet.org/Reports/2012/Cell-Activities. Accessed December 3, 2014.
7. Sarasohn-Kahn J. Participatory health: online and mobile tools help chronically ill manage their care. Oakland (CA): California HealthCare Foundation; 2009.
8. Wood FG, Robson MP, Thompson MK, et al. Selecting the best type of mobile application for diabetes self-management. CIN Plus 2013;31:208–11.
9. American Diabetes Association. Standards of medical care in diabetes. Diabetes Care 2012;35(Suppl 1):s11–63.
10. Centers for Disease Control and Prevention. National Diabetes Surveillance System. Available at: http://gis.cdc.gov/grasp/diabetes/DiabetesAtlas.html. Accessed December 8, 2014.

11. Centers for Disease Control and Prevention. Diabetes Public Health Resource. Available at: http://www.cdc.gov/diabetes/statistics/prevalence_national.htm. Accessed December 8, 2014.

12. Davis TC, Crouch MA, Long SW, et al. Rapid assessment of literacy levels of adult primary care patients. Fam Med 1991;23:433–5.

13. Toobert DJ, Hampson SE, Glasgow RE. The summary of diabetes self-care activities measure: Results from 7 studies and a revised measure. Diabetes Care 2000;23:943–50.

14. Lorig K, Stewart A, Ritter P, et al. Outcome measures for health education and other health care interventions. Thousand Oaks (CA): Sage; 1996.

15. Fitzgerald JT, Anderson RM, Funnell MM, et al. The reliability and validity of a brief diabetes knowledge test. Diabetes Care 1998;21(5):706–10.

Smoking in Rural and Underserved Pregnant Women

Marilyn Cooper Handley, RN, MSN, PhD[a],*,
Daniel M. Avery Jr, MD[b]

KEYWORDS

- Smoking rates • Effects of smoking • Pregnancy • Cessation • Health disparities
- Rural

KEY POINTS

- Although strides have been made in the last 50 years to reduce smoking rates, much more needs to be done.
- Smoking continues to negatively impact the health outcomes of individuals.
- Health disparities and smoking result in exponential health effects.
- Pregnant women and their unborn infants are at extreme risk when smoking during pregnancy.
- Health care providers must address health disparities to reduce the incidence of smoking in pregnant women.

INTRODUCTION OF PROBLEM

More than 50 years have passed since the first Surgeon General's Report on Smoking and Health, yet smoking remains a major contributor to poor health outcomes. Warner (2014)[1] states that despite widespread public education, development of cessation programs, and a general reduction in rates of smoking, smoking continues to be a major health concern. A general state of apathy seems to exist among the general population and health care providers alike. The perceived consensus is that people are aware of the inherent dangers of smoking. An indifferent attitude exists that purports individuals know smoking is bad for their health and that it is futile to attempt to change

The authors do hereby declare that no potential conflict of interest exists. This project was unfunded.
[a] Capstone College of Nursing, University of Alabama, Box 870358, Tuscaloosa, AL 35487-0358, USA; [b] College of Community Health Sciences, University of Alabama, Tuscaloosa, AL, USA
* Corresponding author. Box 870358, Tuscaloosa, AL 35487-0358.
E-mail address: mhandley@ua.edu

that behavior. Indeed, Warner (2014)[1] states a common perception is that smoking is old news and a problem solved. However, smoking continues to be a significant health problem in the general population, contributing to chronic disease, death, and increased health care costs. Smoking is a major behavioral health risk factor in the care of pregnant women. Smoking increases the risks of complications for the woman and her unborn infant. These problems are multiplied when health disparities are an additional factor.[2] Mendelsohn and colleagues[3] describe pregnancy as a window of opportunity for smoking cessation. They think women may be motivated to quit smoking to improve the health of their unborn infant. However, an estimated 16.4% of pregnant smokers in the United States continue to smoke. The purpose of this article is to explore the often-overlooked implications of smoking in the rural and underserved populations, especially pregnant women.

BACKGROUND
Smoking in the General Population

Smoking in the general population has been recognized as a serious health problem. The Surgeon General's Report on Smoking in 1964 reported the causal link between smoking and lung cancer.[4] In the decades since then, research has documented the negative effects of cigarette smoking on human health. Smoking is responsible for approximately 20% of deaths in the United States each year. Many other individuals develop extensive chronic diseases, including cancer, cardiovascular disease, and respiratory disease. Smoking has been associated with complications in reproduction, diabetes, and immune system disorders.[5] Smoking is the most prevalent, yet modifiable risk factor for health and well-being.[5,6] The Surgeon General's Report focused on the harmful effects of smoking on health. Before that time, smoking was socially acceptable and even a status symbol among popular stereotypes. Individuals who smoked were viewed as sophisticated, cool, macho, or sexy. Advertising media used the smoker's image to market products as a means of controlling weight and enhancing glamour, independence, success, and even athleticism.[4]

The 2014 Surgeon General's Report, The Health Consequences of Smoking: 50 Years of Progress,[6] highlights many accomplishments that have been achieved in the effort to reduce smoking. Efforts to educate the public about the dangers of smoking and to facilitate smoking cessation have proliferated. These efforts range from educational pamphlets for individual distribution to widespread media campaigns in magazines and on television. The national rate of adults who smoke has decreased dramatically.[7] A decade ago, smoking was common in most public areas. Progress has been made in the provision of smoke-free public areas, such as restaurants, colleges, sporting events, and public buildings. Now many businesses, colleges, and other public areas are either tobacco free or smoke free. However, in spite of these accomplishments, there remains a core of individuals who continue to smoke. Review of national data from efforts undertaken to track these efforts indicate that the significant proportion of the individuals who smoke are from rural or disadvantaged backgrounds.[7]

Smoking Rates in the United States

The overall rates of individuals who smoke have declined since the Surgeon General's report was issued in 1964, when approximately 42% of adults smoked. The rate decreased significantly by 2005, when the rate reached 20.9%. This rate represented an approximate 50% decrease in the smoking rate over that time period. Since then, the percentage of individuals who smoke has continued to decrease overall; however, the rate of cessation has slowed. The rate of smoking by women has declined much slower than the rates for men.[3] In the 7 years between 2005 and 2012, the overall current smoking rate decreased less than 3.0% to 18.1%. Education has also been a significant predictor in smoking rates. The percentage gap between those with a college education when compared with those with a college education increased from 12.0% for those with lower educational levels in 1964 to a 29.2% gap between educational levels in 2011.[1] These rates highlight those core groups who continue to smoke and experience a disproportionate rate of complications from smoking.

Health Consequences or Effects of Smoking

The effects of health disparities are evident in many areas of health care. These effects are particularly impressive when one looks at disparities and smoking. Health disparities are defined in the report from Healthy People 2010[8] as "a particular type of health difference that is closely linked with social, economic, and/or environmental disadvantage."[8] Other definitions have been offered; however, they all speak to the link between demographics and negative health outcomes. Disparities include a variety of factors, often mentioned are racial/ethnic group, women, physical or mental impairments, and rural dwellers. The importance of considering health disparities highlights the strong, multifactorial relationships that exist between health, genetics, behaviors, health services, socioeconomic status, literacy, and population groups. James[9] reports on the changing demography of the rural United States. He cites determinants such as use of self-care, regular source of care, lifestyle behaviors, poverty, higher rates of female-led households, income inequality, and unique cultural differences as examples of individual, structural, or contextual levels of health disparities.

Cigarette smoking continues to negatively affect the quality and cost of health in the United States.[4] Warner[1] cites smoking as the prime cause of lung and laryngeal cancer, chronic bronchitis, coronary heart disease, and emphysema. McAfee[4] reports that complications from smoking have risen sharply in women and are now equal to the rates in men for lung cancer, chronic obstructive pulmonary disease (COPD), and cardiovascular diseases. Smoking has been linked to breast cancer, colorectal cancer, and liver cancer. Research has also shown that smoking is linked with higher rates of recurrence of cancer and poorer responses to treatment. Risks of dying from aneurysms, stroke, and heart attack are higher for women who smoke than for male smokers. Women who smoke also experience a disproportionate rate of respiratory complications. COPD, emphysema, bronchitis, and asthma are all increased in women who smoke.[3]

Smoking rates and the negative health effects of smoking hit hardest on individuals in health-disparity classifications. Educational level is a significant factor as the rate of smoking increases inversely with a decrease in education. The Campaign for Tobacco-Free Kids states rates of smoking are directly correlated with years of education and income level. Rates of smoking are inversely related to socioeconomic status with those living at less than the poverty level having a rate 11% higher than those living at or greater than the poverty level. Smoking rates are lower in the West and Northeast as opposed to the Midwest and South where many individuals live in rural areas. The highest reported rate is found in Kentucky at 28%. This higher rate of smoking in the South and Midwest is likely linked to a combination of lower education and economic levels. The age group with the highest rate of smoking is between 25 and 44 years of age.[10] The percentage rate among different racial/ethnic groups is interesting because of the lower rates of smoking in Asian and Hispanic groups. Non-Hispanic whites and blacks, American Indians, Alaska Natives, and individuals of multiple races have the highest rates ranging between 18.1% and 26.1%[4] (**Table 1**).

Table 1		
Percentage of adult smokers in 2012		
By sex	Adult men	20.5%
	Adult women	15.8%
By age	18–24 y	17.3%
	25–44 y	21.6%
	45–64 y	19.5%
	65 y and older	8.9%
By race/ethnicity	Multiple-race individuals	26.1%
	American Indians/Alaska Natives (non-Hispanic)	21.8%
	Whites (non-Hispanic)	19.7%
	Blacks (non-Hispanic)	18.1%
	Hispanics	12.5%
	Asians (non-Hispanic; excludes Native Hawaiians & Pacific Islanders)	10.7%
By education	Adults with a GED diploma	41.9%
	Adults with 12 or less years of education (no diploma)	24.7%
	Adults with a high school diploma	23.1%
	Adults with an undergraduate college degree	9.1%
	Adults with a postgraduate college degree	5.9%
Poverty status	Adults who live at less than the poverty level	27.9%
	Adults who live at or greater than the poverty level	17.0%
US total	Current smokers (represents about 42.1 million Americans)	18.1%

Abbreviation: GED, general equivalency diploma.
Data from McAfee T, Burnette D. The impact of smoking on women's health. J Womens Health 2014;23(11):881–5.

Reductions in smoking rates have shown improvement in health status for many. However, these gains have not been shared by all. Villarruel[11] spoke of an "intersectionality among race, ethnicity, gender, and social class" that negatively influences health. In summary, the poorer and less educated, with lower incomes, are the ones more likely to smoke and experience the negative health effects. Those with less access to care and less social support are less likely to attempt or follow through with cessation programs.[1] The negative effects of smoking are overwhelmingly borne by those less able to seek care.

CESSATION METHODS AND PROGRAMS

Many smoking cessation programs abound and are generally available to individuals who seek them. These programs or strategies range from those aimed at society in general, such as higher prices, smoke-free regulations, mass media campaigns to state and local programs that provide education, and/or medications to individuals.[3] Most seek to provide barrier-free access by providing education and medications at no or reduced cost. Mendelsohn and colleagues[3] state that, although nicotine replacement therapy can be used in pregnancy, behavioral counseling is the first-line of treatment. Barriers to smoking cessation, especially during pregnancy, cluster around several health disparities. The Healthy People 2010[8] report cited a lack of resources, transportation, decreased health care coverage, lack of sufficient income to pay for care, lack of informational sources related to smoking and cessation programs, and decreased access to providers as major barriers to smoking cessation. Correll and colleagues[10] cite lower educational levels and decreased medical resources and cessation assistance as factors influencing smoking in southern rural dwellers.

Many of the cessation interventions in health care involve a process similar to the 5 As. The 5 As are steps in the systematic approach and care of individuals who smoke. The As represent ask, advise, assess, assist, and arrange. When followed, the individual is asked about readiness to stop smoking; advised of the risk; smoking habits are assessed; assistance is given in the form of tips to help quit; and finally, arrangements are made for follow-up (often with cessation programs). The 5 As are recommended for use by providers by the Association of Women's Health, Obstetric, and Neonatal Nurses and the American College of Obstetricians and Gynecologists[12,13] (**Box 1**).

WOMEN AND SMOKING

Smoking results in unique medical concerns for women and their infants. These concerns begin during pregnancy and continue into the neonatal period and early childhood. The untoward effects are manifested predominately in the serious conditions of prematurity and low birth weight. Approximately 1 in 6 women smoke cigarettes. Reasons for smoking include weight control, peer pressure, depression, stress, and rebellion against authority figures, such as parents. Women with the lowest educational levels are most likely to smoke.[10] Ethnic differences show the highest rates of women who smoke are in the American Indian and Alaskan populations, followed by Caucasian and African American women. The lowest rates of smoking in women are seen in Hispanic and Asian women. The Surgeon General's Report from 1980 recognized that women experience different health effects from smoking possibly because of sex differences and genetics. Smoking in women has been associated with respiratory conditions, such as lung cancer, COPD, emphysema, and bronchitis; cardiovascular diseases, such as coronary artery disease, stroke, aneurysms, and peripheral vascular disease; and complications related to pregnancy.[10]

SMOKING IN PREGNANCY

The pregnant smoker is at an increased risk for poor pregnancy outcomes in addition to the risks to her health. Risks include chronic cardiovascular and respiratory complications and hemorrhage related to placental conditions. The woman's risks for poor pregnancy outcomes for the newborn include preterm birth, low birth weight, hypoxia, stillbirth, and neonatal death.[10,14] Low birth weight has been identified as a leading cause of neonatal morbidity and mortality in the United States. The incidence of low

---

Box 1
5 As to smoking cessation

Ask: Individuals should be asked about smoking status at each health care encounter.

Advise: Each individual who smokes should be provided with information about why they should quit smoking.

Assess: Individuals' readiness to quit should be assessed. Health care providers should explore reasons for smoking in order to offer specific suggestions and identify barriers.

Assist: The health care provider is seen as a trusted advisor. They are in unique positions to provide suggestions, tips, and other resources.

Arrange: Referring to a cessation program, providing information about referrals, and setting a quit date are all ways the health care provider may encourage an individual to stop smoking.

birth weight is positively related to the mother's smoking status and the number of cigarettes smoked per day. Smoking in pregnancy results in an overwhelming burden of cost to the individuals and to society. Although the reduction of low birth weight was a goal of Healthy People 2010, little progress was made. Reduction of low birth weight is once again a goal of Healthy People 2020.[8] Smoking is the major health behavior negatively linked to low birth weight and prematurity. However, there is hope as smoking cessation during pregnancy has been shown to reduce the risk of complications.[3]

Studies have shown that a small percentage of pregnant women will stop smoking when pregnant, but most pregnant women who smoke continue with severe risks for themselves and their unborn infants.[3,15] This circumstance is especially true in the South and in younger, less-educated, and otherwise disadvantaged populations. Lower economic levels and access to care are frequently identified as factors that contribute to fewer individuals enrolling in smoking cessation efforts.[16]

RISKS ASSOCIATED WITH SMOKING IN PREGNANCY

Smoking negatively affects the cardiovascular and respiratory systems of the individual who smokes. In pregnant women, the effects on the vascular system predispose the woman to difficulties with conception, higher rates of miscarriage, and fetal anomalies, especially cleft lip and palate. Vascular complications put the woman at an increased risk of hemorrhagic problems, such as placenta previa and hemorrhage. The operative delivery rate is higher for women who smoke than for those who do not. This higher rate is often caused by nonreassuring heart rates of the fetus during labor (presumably from decreased oxygen through the placenta to the fetus). The women who smoke during pregnancy are significantly more likely to experience preterm labor and birth and infants who are born prematurely. They are also more likely to have infants die during the first year of life. Smoking during pregnancy contributes to a high financial burden for care. The American Lung Association reported the costs related to preterm infants born to women who smoked during pregnancy exceeded $350 million each year. The March of Dimes reported that in 2005, preterm birth in the United States resulted in a societal economic annual cost of at least $26.2 billion. This figure included medical, educational, and lost productivity costs related to preterm infants.[17]

The infant morbidity and mortality rates are higher for infants born to women in rural areas and those with lower educational and income levels. These groups are more likely to smoke than their counterparts. These facts support Villarreal's[11] statement of intersectionality of demographic factors negatively influencing health outcomes. Reported reasons to smoke include weight control, stress control, and social situations where others smoke. The list of negative effects of smoking on the health of women,[18] especially during pregnancy, is staggering, particularly when one realizes the outcomes could be changed.

SUMMARY

The risks of smoking in pregnancy, especially in rural and underserved women dealing with health disparities, must be aggressively addressed by health care providers. This increased focus must include a heightened awareness among providers of the risks and the potential for improved outcomes. The implementation of best practices related to smoking cessation could significantly reduce the percentage of women who smoke and improve pregnancy outcomes. Every woman should be asked about her smoking status and advised of the health risks; her willingness to quit should be assessed; she should be given assistance in the form of counseling and/or medications to assist her to quit; and follow-up within the health care site or with external organizations must be arranged. The literature has shown that individuals usually try to stop smoking several times before they are successful. Clinically focused strategies should emphasize understanding why the individual smokes and address cessation with interventions tailored to meet the individual needs. Health care providers must take a fresh look at the problem and seek to understand the factors related to those who continue to smoke, especially during pregnancy. A broader recommendation would be for community agencies to develop programs related to stress reduction and adaptation to parenting. Identified areas for consideration include education and resource referrals to reduce or remove barriers to smoking cessation and enhance parenting. Research must explore the understanding of barriers to health behavior change in rural and underserved populations to better incorporate education and appropriate interventions to improve cessation rates in those who smoke, especially during pregnancy.

REFERENCES

1. Warner KE. Editorial: 50 years since the first Surgeon General's report on smoking and health: a happy anniversary? Am J Public Health 2014;104(1):5–8.
2. Levis DM, Stone-Wiggins B, O'Hegarty M, et al. Women's perspectives on smoking and pregnancy and graphic warning labels. Am J Health Behav 2014;38(5): 755–64.
3. Mendelsohn C, Gould GS, Oncken C. Management of smoking in pregnant women. Aust Fam Physician 2014;43(1):46–51.
4. McAfee T, Burnette D. The impact of smoking on women's health. J Women's Health (Larchmt) 2014;23(11):881–5.
5. Center for Disease Control and Prevention: Adult cigarette smoking in the United States: current estimates. Available at: www.cdc.gov/tobacco/data_statistics/ fact_sheets/adult_data/cig_smoking/index.htm#. Accessed December 8, 2014.
6. HHS. The health consequences of smoking - 50 years of progress: a report of the Surgeon General, 2014. Available at: http://www.surgeongeneral.gov/library/ reports/50-years-of-progress/. Accessed September 15, 2014.
7. CDC: Health effects of cigarette smoking. Smoking & tobacco use. Available at: http://www.cdc.gov/tobacco/data_statistics/fact_sheets/health_effects/effects_ cigsmoking/#overview. Accessed December 18, 2014.
8. Healthy People.gov Disparities Available at: http://www.healthypeople.gov/2020/ about/foundation_health_measures/Disparities. Accessed December 14, 2014.
9. James WL. All rural places are not created equal: revisiting the rural mortality penalty in the United States. Am J Public Health 2014;104(11):2122–9.
10. Correll JA, Dalton WT, Bailey B. Weight concerns, body image, and smoking continuation in pregnant women in rural Appalachia. Am J Health Behav 2013; 37(6):734–44.
11. Villarruel AM. Health disparities research: issues, strategies, and innovations. J Multicultural Nurs Health 2006;12(1):4–9.
12. Chang JC, Alexander SC, Holland CL, et al. Smoking is bad for babies: obstetric care providers' use of best practice smoking cessation counseling techniques. Am J Health Promot 2013;27(3):170–6.
13. Albrecht SA. Smoking cessation in pregnancy. Nurs Womens Health 2010;14(3): 177–9.
14. Amasha, Hadayat A, Jaradeh, et al. Effect of active and passive smoking during pregnancy on its outcomes. Health Sci J 2012;6(2):335–52.

15. Masho SW, Bishop DL, Keyser-Marcus L, et al. Least explored factors associated with prenatal smoking. Matern Child Health J 2013;17:1167–74.
16. Page RL, Padilla YC, Hamilton ER. Psychosocial factors associated with patterns of smoking surrounding pregnancy in fragile families. Matern Child Health J 2012; 16:249–57.
17. March of Dimes PeriStats perinatal overview. Available at: www.marchofdimes. org/Peristats/pdflib/999/pds_01_all.pdf. Accessed December 8, 2014.
18. Hershberger P. Smoking and pregnant teens. Lifelines 1998;2(4):26–31.

The Presence of Risk Factors for Type 2 Diabetes Mellitus in Underserved Preschool Children

 CrossMark

Michele Montgomery, PhD, MPH, RN[a],*, Paige Johnson, PhD, RN[a],
Patrick Ewell, MA[b]

KEYWORDS

- Preschool children • African Americans • Type 2 diabetes mellitus
- Health screening • Risk factors

KEY POINTS

- Obesity and increasing rates of type 2 diabetes mellitus in children is a public health concern.
- Medically underserved, minority children are at risk for the development of type 2 diabetes mellitus.
- The most common risk factors for the development of type 2 diabetes mellitus in this population of minority children are family history of diabetes mellitus, elevated body mass index, and elevated blood pressure.

INTRODUCTION

Type 2 diabetes mellitus (T2DM) is a public health priority in the United States because of its high prevalence and its negative long-term impact on health.[1] Once considered only a problem among adults, the prevalence of T2DM in children is rapidly increasing in the United States.[2,3]

The prevalence of T2DM is expected to quadruple by the year 2050, with youths of minority race/ethnic groups being primarily affected.[4]

In the United States, high prevalence rates for T2DM ($\geq$10.6%) exist in a distinct geographic pattern, which is referred to as the *diabetes belt*. West Virginia, the

Disclosures: The authors have no actual or potential conflict of interests that need to be disclosed.
[a] Capstone College of Nursing, The University of Alabama, Box 870358, Tuscaloosa, AL 35487, USA; [b] Department of Psychology, The University of Alabama, Box 870348, Tuscaloosa, AL 35487-0348, USA
* Corresponding author. Capstone College of Nursing, The University of Alabama, Box 870358, Tuscaloosa, AL 35487.
E-mail address: mmontgomery1@ua.edu

Appalachian counties of Tennessee and Kentucky, much of the Mississippi Delta, and a southern belt extending across Louisiana, Mississippi, middle Alabama, south Georgia, and the coastal regions of the Carolinas[5] are included in the diabetes belt area (**Fig. 1**). It is thought that higher rates of T2DM exist in this specific geographic pattern because of the prevailing social norms, community and environmental factors, socioeconomic status, and genetic risk factors.[6]

County Perspective

Tuscaloosa County, which is located in western Alabama, is included in the diabetes belt with a prevalence of T2DM of 11%.[7] Several risk factors put residents of this county at risk for developing T2DM, including high rates of obesity and physical inactivity, race, socioeconomic status, and lack of access to healthy foods.[7] Approximately 30% of residents are African American; 25.5% live in a rural area; 18% report food insecurity; 7% report limited access to healthy foods; 19% of adults and 4% of children are uninsured; 33% of adults are obese; and 28% report physical inactivity. Although national databases exist that characterize diabetes at the national and state levels,[1] studies are needed at the local level where health-promotion interventions will ultimately be designed and implemented. Studies conducted at the local level that focus on identifying individuals at risk for developing T2DM, particularly children, will enable more efficient prevention policies and programs to be implemented in an effort to reduce the prevalence of diabetes.

RISK FACTORS FOR TYPE 2 DIABETES MELLITUS IN CHILDREN

The primary risk factors for the development of T2DM in children include obesity, ethnicity, family history of diabetes, and the presence of insulin resistance.[8,9] Obesity has been identified as the major risk factor for the development of T2DM in children,[3,8]

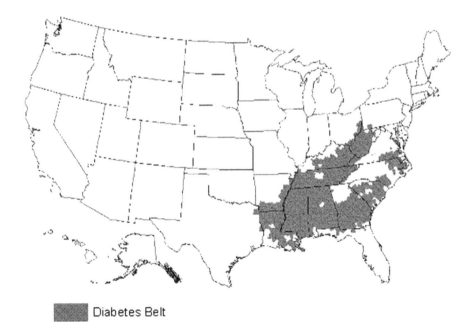

Diabetes Belt

Fig. 1. Diabetes belt. (*From* Centers for Disease Control. CDC identifies diabetes belt. Available at: http://www.cdc.gov/diabetes/pdfs/newsroom/diabetesbelt.pdf. Accessed April 29, 2015.)

and T2DM is one of the leading causes of death in the United States and among the medically underserved residents of Alabama.[10,11] Childhood obesity continues to be a significant public health concern, with the prevalence of obesity among preschool-aged children most recently estimated at 8.4%.[12] Many states showed downward trends in obesity among low-income, preschool-aged children.[13] However, the prevalence of obesity among this age group in Alabama actually increased from 13.8% in 2008 to 14.1% in 2011. According to the Centers for Disease Control and Prevention (CDC), preschoolers who are identified as overweight or obese are 5 times more likely to become overweight or obese adults in comparison with their nonobese peers.[14,15]

There are also geographic, racial, and income disparities associated with obesity in rural dwellers, African Americans, and residents of lower socioeconomic status. This finding is especially troubling considering the risk of developing T2DM is greater among ethnic minorities, such as African American, Hispanic, Asian American, Pacific Islander, Native American, and Alaska Native children compared with non-Hispanic whites.[16] Therefore, obesity further increases their risk for developing this disease.

Most children diagnosed with T2DM have a family history of diabetes.[17,18] According to the American Diabetes Association (ADA), 40% to 80% of children diagnosed with T2DM had one parent with T2DM, and 74% to 90% reported having at least one first- or second-degree relative diagnosed with T2DM.[3]

Obesity is also associated with insulin resistance and hyperinsulinemia, which are hallmark symptoms of T2DM. Because of the excess adipose tissue, obese children produce too much insulin, which leads to insulin resistance and compensatory hyperinsulemia.[18] Insulin resistance and hyperinsulinemia are not easily assessed in children. However, clinical indicators that can be assessed include acanthosis nigricans, hypertension, and dyslipidemia.[17–19] Acanthosis nigricans (AN) is a hyperpigmentation and thickening of the skin folds at the back of the neck, axillae, and medial aspects of the thighs. AN has been well documented as a clinical indicator of hyperinsulinemia and is associated with insulin resistance.[20] It has been reported that 60% to 90% of children with T2DM have AN.[8]

Comorbidities associated with both obesity and insulin resistance include hypertension and dyslipidemia. Children between 1 and 17 years of age whose blood pressure readings are between the 90th and 95th percentile for age, sex, and height are considered prehypertensive and, therefore, at risk for developing hypertension.[21] Hypertension is defined as an average systolic blood pressure or diastolic blood pressure that is greater than or equal to the 95th percentile for sex, age, and height on at least 3 separate occasions.

Dyslipidemia, which is abnormally high lipids or lipoproteins in the blood, is another clinical indicator of insulin resistance and hyperinsulinemia. Dyslipidemia is also associated with obesity, and previous studies have demonstrated strong relationships between blood lipid levels and anthropometry in preschool and school-aged children.[22–25] Two particularly consistent relationships are the association of increased height with a more favorable blood lipid profile and of obesity with a less favorable blood lipid profile among children. The National Heart, Lung, and Blood Institute recommends total cholesterol values remain less than 170 mg/dL in children and adolescents aged 2 to 19 years and consider any value greater than 200 mg/dL to be high.[21]

SCREENING
Screening Initiative

In 2004, a consensus panel convened by the ADA published recommendations for screening in children.[26] Appropriate screening of preschool children can be expected to result in earlier identification of those children at risk for the development of T2DM, and early screening programs can help reduce the risk of complications. Although there may be concern that screenings outside of the health care setting may not be effective because of failure of parents to seek follow-up testing, school-based screenings can be beneficial in screening a large group of children who may otherwise not receive screening.

The Tuscaloosa Pre-K Initiative is a collaborative preschool program that was established in 2007 to reach all 4-year-old children in the City of Tuscaloosa deemed academically at risk and provide them with the best health and education services possible. The Pre-K Initiative is a 9-month preschool program that prepares children to enter kindergarten while providing comprehensive family support services and programs. As part of the support services and because this population of children may not receive routine health checkups, yearly health screenings are a required component of the Pre-K Initiative and have an 85% to 95% student participation rate. Routinely, the school nurses monitor the follow-up by parents when children are identified as having an immediate unmet health need. However, no comprehensive analysis of the data collected from 2007 to 2014 was conducted to identify risk factors for diabetes in this population.

Purpose

This analysis was a secondary data analysis to determine the presence of selected risk factors for the development of T2DM (high-risk racial/ethnic group, obesity, elevated blood pressure, elevated casual blood glucose, elevated total cholesterol, and the presence of AN) in underserved preschool children in Tuscaloosa, Alabama with or without a family history of diabetes. The research questions are as follows: (1) What is the prevalence of risk factors for T2DM among preschool children enrolled in the Pre-K Initiative? (2) What is the incidence of selected T2DM risk factors in preschool children with a positive family history of diabetes? (3) What is the relationship between each of the selected risk factors and a positive family history of T2DM?

METHODS
Participants

This sample consisted of 1019 (505 boys) preschool children between 4 and 5 years of age who were enrolled in a public school system preschool program (Pre-K Initiative). This sample was collected from health fairs, conducted as a part of the Pre-K Initiative, during a 6-year period between January 2007 and January 2014. Of the participants sampled, 84.5% were African American, 8.6% Hispanic, 4.6% Caucasian, and 2.4% American Indian, Asian, or other.

The secondary data analysis sought to identify preschool children who would be representative of minority children from low socioeconomic families in the state of Alabama. A single public school system was chosen in order to capture a representative sample of the target population. All children enrolled in the preschool program were provided the opportunity to participate in the school health fairs. Only students who had parental consent were permitted to participate in the health fairs and were included in this study. The Institutional Review Board of the university system and the city school system provided approval for the study.

Procedure

Physical assessments were performed at on-site health fairs conducted at 9 preschools located in disadvantaged areas around the city. The health fairs were organized into a series of health assessment stations that included vital signs, finger stick, head-to-toe examination, vision screening, and hearing screening. City school personnel, preschool teachers, school nurses, and nursing students and faculty organized the health fair. At the vital signs station, height, weight, blood pressure, respirations, and pulse were obtained. The casual blood glucose and total cholesterol were obtained at the finger-stick station, and results were recorded on the health assessment form. Children who exhibited any risk factor results beyond the normal parameters were referred to their primary health care provider.

Measures

A health assessment form was used to document the results of the screenings conducted at the school health fairs. This information included results of vital signs (eg, height, weight, and blood pressure), a brief head-to-toe physical examination that included inspecting for the presence of AN, casual (nonfasting) blood glucose, and total cholesterol.

Body mass index (BMI) was calculated using the CDC's Children's BMI Tool for Schools.[27] The Children's BMI Tool for Schools is a Excel (Microsoft Corporation, Redmond, WA, USA) spreadsheet intended for use by school, child care, and other professionals who want to compute BMI based on age for a group of up to 2000 children. For example, this tool could be used for a school classroom or entire grade of students. This calculator computes BMI and BMI percentiles for individual children in a group using height and weight measurements, sex, date of birth, and date of measurement information that is entered. Any student with a BMI-for-age in the 85th percentile or greater was classified as at risk for being overweight or obese. Blood pressure was measured using an appropriately sized pediatric cuff. Evaluation of the blood pressure reading was based on the child's sex, age, and height. Any child who was considered prehypertensive using the guidelines set forth by the National High Blood Pressure Education Program Working Group on Children and Adolescents[28] for childhood blood pressure was deemed at risk. The casual blood glucose and total cholesterol were obtained by performing a finger stick on the child. Casual blood glucose and total cholesterol levels of 200 mg/dL or greater were considered elevated.

Data Analysis

Descriptive and inferential statistics were used to evaluate the study data. Descriptive statistics (ie, frequencies and measures of central tendencies) were used to analyze the demographic data. Prevalence of risk factors for T2DM was determined for the entire sample population based on the guidelines stated earlier. Seven risk factors were investigated, including ethnic background, family history, BMI, blood pressure, cholesterol, glucose level, and presence of AN. Inferential statistics were used to assess for variations in children with a presence or absence of family history of diabetes. The presence of risk factors was evaluated for both groups using an independent t-test. Finally, risk factors were related to possible outcome variables. Chi-square was used to examine the relationship between selected risk factors for T2DM in children with or without a family history of diabetes.

RESULTS
Participant Profile

Profile of type 2 diabetes risk factors

Individuals with 2 or more risk factors have a greater chance of developing T2DM.[9] A total of 601 children (59%) screened in this study presented with 2 or more of the identified risk factors for T2DM. The cumulative number of risk factors for children who participated in the health fair can be found in **Table 1**.

Table 1
Sums and percentages of total risk factors

No. of Risk Factors	N (%)
0	78 (7.7)
1	340 (33.4)
2	368 (36.1)
3	191 (18.7)
4	40 (3.9)
5	2 (0.2)

Because this study sought to investigate a group of minority, underserved children, most (87.4%) of the children in the present study had an ethnic background that would cause them to be considered at risk. Other than ethnicity, the most commonly identified risk factors in this sample were family history of diabetes (31.4%), overweight/obesity (31.1%), and elevated blood pressure (24.9%). Although elevated cholesterol and glucose and signs of AN are risk factors for T2DM, these were not identified in this sample population. A complete list of risk factors can be found in **Table 2**.

As stated earlier, positive family history for diabetes was reported by 31% of the total sample. **Table 3** shows the incidence of selected T2DM risk factors for those children with and without a family history of diabetes. An independent t-test showed that when family history was excluded from total risk factors, those who had a family history of diabetes ($M = 1.59$, $SD = .78$) had significantly ($t[1017] = -3.18$, $P = .002$) more risk factors than those who had no family history ($M = 1.41$, $SD = .83$).

Most of the participants were considered at risk because of ethnic background; therefore, the number of risk factors was calculated excluding ethnicity (**Table 4**). Once ethnicity was eliminated, 245 children (24.0%) presented with 2 or more risk factors, and 38.3% had at least one risk factor.

This sample was also divided by sex to look for differences in risk factors. Boys were more likely to be at risk for blood pressure (chi-square $[X^2] = 26.97$, $P<.002$; **Table 5**) and had more total risk factors than girls ($t[1017] = 2.15$, $P = .032$).

In this sample, the number of total doctor visits within the last year was also collected. This variable serves a possible outcome variable to assess health risk because those children who go to the doctor more are more likely to have poorer health and greater health care cost. Each risk factor was used as a predictor variable and regressed onto the total number of doctor visits in the last year. The number of doctor visits was significantly related to both BMI ($\beta = 0.12$, $t[828] = 3.49$,

Table 2
Prevalence of each risk factor

	Not at Risk N (%)	At Risk N (%)
Ethnic	128 (12.6)	891 (87.4)
Family history	699 (68.6)	320 (31.4)
BMI	702 (68.9)	317 (31.1)
Blood pressure	765 (75.1)	254 (24.9)
Cholesterol	989 (97.1)	30 (2.9)
AN	1015 (99.6)	4 (0.4)
Glucose	1016 (99.6)	3 (0.3)

Table 3
Chi-square division of family history compared with ethnic background and BMI

	Not at Risk Because of FH, N (%)	At Risk Because of FH, N (%)	X^2 (P)
Ethnic at risk	586 (66.9)	295 (33.1)	9.58 (.002)
Ethnic not at risk	103 (80.5)	25 (19.5)	—
BMI at risk	201 (63.4)	116 (36.6)	5.75 (.016)
BMI not at risk	498 (70.9)	204 (29.1)	—

Closer investigation via chi-square shows that those with a family history were more likely to be at risk because of BMI (X^2 = 17.82, P<.001) and because of ethnic background (X^2 = 9.59, P = .002).
Abbreviations: FH, family history; X^2, chi-square.

P = .001) and family history of diabetes (β = 0.07, t[828] = 2.07, P = .039) indicating that both of these risk factors may lead to more doctor visits.

DISCUSSION

According to the ADA, T2DM accounts for approximately 45% of diabetes diagnosed in children in the United States depending on geographic region and ethnicity.[3] Because of this growing epidemic, the ADA established screening criteria that can be used to identify children at risk for the development of T2DM. Being overweight or obese and the presence of 2 or more risk factors (ie, family history, ethnicity, signs of insulin resistance) place children at an increased risk for the development of T2DM. Childhood obesity is a growing public health concern and is more common among low-income and minority children. Because obesity is very likely to track into adulthood, prevention of obesity is much more effective than treating obesity once it is established; early identification of overweight or obese children may assist with implementing effective interventions. Thirty-one percent of the students screened had a BMI greater than the 85th percentile for age and sex, and this finding exceeds national and state statistics on overweight and obesity in preschool children.

It has previously been reported that family history is a commonly identified risk factor for the development of T2DM.[8,26,29] According to Kaufman,[8] 45% to 80% of children who develop T2DM have a parent with T2DM. In the authors' study, 31% of children screened had a positive family history of diabetes.

This study also compared the risk profile of a group of low-income, minority children with and without a family history of diabetes. Those who had a family history of diabetes had significantly more risk factors than those who had no family history and were more likely to be at risk because of BMI and ethnicity. This finding is in contrast to a previous study that examined T2DM risk factors in a group of rural schoolchildren

Table 4
Sums and percentages of total risk factors excluding ethnic background

No. of Risk Factors	N (%)
0	384 (37.7)
1	390 (38.3)
2	199 (19.5)
3	44 (4.3)
4	2 (0.2)

Table 5
Chi-square division of sex compared with blood pressure

	Males N (%)	Females N (%)	X^2 (P)
Blood pressure at risk	157 (61.8)	97 (38.2)	26.97 (.002)
Blood pressure not at risk	348 (46.2)	367 (48.7)	—

between 5 and 21 years of age and reported that those children with no family history of diabetes had more risk factors than those with a family history.[30]

Limitations

Limitations of this study include missing information on the parent survey or health assessment forms. The parent survey required self-reported information, and family history of diabetes may not have been accurately reported. Some children may have missed stations at the health fair or their parents may have only given permission for limited health screenings, so some information may have been missing from the health assessment forms. Nonparticipants in the health fair screenings may represent a higher-risk subgroup. Therefore, risk factors in this medically underserved population of preschool children may be underestimated. A final limitation addresses the generalizability of the study findings. The ethnic makeup of the study population exceeds national percentages for African American populations[31]; therefore, they may not be generalizable to other groups.

Implications for Clinical Practice

This study helped identify the importance of early screening for diabetes in low-income, minority preschool children. Because of the microvascular and macrovascular damage to organs, T2DM can have a significant impact on the health, quality of life, and health care costs over a lifetime. This impact is especially significant for those developing the disease at an early age; thus, early identification of those at risk is imperative to improving the long-term health of children.

Because these children often may not receive yearly checkups or have a regular health care provider, conducting these screenings in the school setting can be particularly helpful. In addition, health care providers may perform body measurements during clinic visits but may not have time to sufficiently analyze the results in order to identify at-risk children who need further intervention. Nurses are in an ideal position to educate parents regarding dietary changes, physical activity, and the importance of weight management and to help them understand the potential long-term impact the identified risk factors can make on the health of their child.

REFERENCES

1. Centers for Disease Control and Prevention. State-specific incidence of diabetes among adults - participating states, 1995-1997 and 2005-2007. MMWR Morb Mortal Wkly Rep 2008;57(43):1169–73.
2. Fagot-Campagna A, Pettitt DJ, Engelgau MM, et al. Type 2 diabetes among North American children and adolescents: an epidemiologic review and a public health perspective. J Pediatr 2000;136(5):664–72.
3. American Diabetes Association. Type 2 diabetes in children and adolescents. Diabetes Care 2000;23(3):381–9.

4. Imperatore G, Boyle JP, Thompson TJ, et al. Projections of type 1 and type 2 diabetes burden in the U.S. population aged <20 years through 2050: dynamic modeling of incidence, mortality, and population growth. Diabetes Care 2012; 35(12):2515–20.

5. Centers for Disease Control and Prevention. Estimated county-level prevalence of diabetes and obesity - United States, 2007. MMWR Morb Mortal Wkly Rep 2009; 58(45):1259–63.

6. Centers for Disease Control and Prevention. Recommended community strategies and measurements to prevent obesity in the United States. MMWR Morb Mortal Wkly Rep 2009;58(No. RR-7):1–26.

7. Robert Wood Johnson Foundation. County health rankings and roadmaps. Updated 2014. Available at: http://www.countyhealthrankings.org/. Accessed October 22, 2014.

8. Kaufman FR. Type 2 diabetes mellitus in children and youth: a new epidemic. J Pediatr Endocrinol Metab 2002;15(Suppl 2):737–44.

9. American Diabetes Association. Standards of medical care in diabetes - 2010. Diabetes Care 2010;33(Suppl 1):S11–61.

10. Roger VL, Go AS, Lloyd-Jones DM, et al. Heart disease and stroke statistics–2011 update: a report from the American Heart Association. Circulation 2011; 123(4):e18–209.

11. National Institute of Diabetes and Digestive and Kidney Diseases. National diabetes statistics, 2011. Available at: http://diabetes.niddk.nih.gov/dm/pubs/statistics/#fast. Accessed February 3, 2014.

12. Ogden CL, Carroll MD, Kit BK, et al. Prevalence of childhood and adult obesity in the united states, 2011-2012. JAMA 2014;311(8):806–14.

13. Centers for Disease Control and Prevention. Vital signs: obesity among low-income, preschool-aged children-united states, 2008-2011. MMWR Morb Mortal Wkly Rep 2013;62(30):629–34.

14. Whitaker RC, Wright JA, Pepe MS, et al. Predicting obesity in young adulthood from childhood and parental obesity. N Engl J Med 1997;337:869–73.

15. Centers for Disease Control and Prevention. Vital signs: obesity among low-income, preschool-aged children-United States. Updated 2011. Available at: http://www.cdc.gov/mmwr/preview/mmwrhtml/mm6231a4.htm. Accessed October 17, 2014.

16. Centers for Disease Control and Prevention. National diabetes fact sheet: national estimates and general information on diabetes and prediabetes in the United States, 2011. Atlanta (GA): US. Department of Health and Human Services, Centers for Disease Control and Prevention; 2011.

17. National Diabetes Education Program. Overview of diabetes in children and adolescents. Updated 2014. Available at: http://www.ndep.nih.gov/media/Overview-of-Diabetes-Children-508_2014.pdf. Accessed December 3, 2014.

18. Copeland KC, Becker D, Gottschalk M, et al. Type 2 diabetes in children and adolescents: risk factors, diagnosis, and treatment. Clin Diabetes 2005;23(4): 181–5.

19. Brosnan CA, Upchurch S, Schreiner B. Type 2 diabetes in children and adolescents: an emerging disease. J Pediatr Health Care 2001;15(4):187–93.

20. Dietz WH. Overweight and precursors of type 2 diabetes mellitus in children and adolescents. J Pediatr 2001;138(4):453–4.

21. National Heart, Lung, and Blood Institute. The fourth report on the diagnosis, evaluation, and treatment of high blood pressure in children and adolescents. Pediatrics 2005;114(2):ii.

22. Rona RJ, Qureshi S, Chinn S. Factors related to total cholesterol and blood pressure in British 9 year olds. J Epidemiol Community Health 1996;50(5):512–8.
23. Forrester TE, Wilks RJ, Bennett FI, et al. Fetal growth and cardiovascular risk factors in Jamaican schoolchildren. BMJ 1996;312(7024):156–60.
24. DeStefano F, Berg RL, Griese GG Jr. Determinants of serum lipid and lipoprotein concentrations in children. Epidemiology 1995;6(4):446–9.
25. Burgos MS, Burgos LT, Camargo MD, et al. Relationship between anthropometric measures and cardiovascular risk factors in children and adolescents. Arq Bras Cardiol 2013;101(4):288–96.
26. American Diabetes Association. Screening for type 2 diabetes. Diabetes Care 2004;27(supp11):S11–4.
27. Centers for Disease Control and Prevention. Children's BMI tool for schools - assessing your weight: children's BMI tool for schools. 2011. Available at: http://www.cdc.gov/healthyweight/assessing/bmi/childrens_BMI/tool_for_schools.html. Accessed October 10, 2014.
28. National High Blood Pressure Education Program Working Group on High Blood Pressure in Children and Adolescents. The fourth report on the diagnosis, evaluation, and treatment of high blood pressure in children and adolescents. Pediatrics 2004;114(2):555–76.
29. Urrutia-Rojas X, Menchaca J. Prevalence of risk for type 2 diabetes in school children. J Sch Health 2006;76(5):189–94.
30. Adams MH, Lammon CA. The presence of family history and the development of type 2 diabetes mellitus risk factors in rural children. J Sch Nurs 2007;23(5):259–66.
31. U.S. Census Bureau. State and county quick facts. Updated 2014. Available at: http://quickfacts.census.gov/qfd/states/00000.html. Accessed December 11, 2014.

Using Mobile Technologies to Access Evidence-Based Resources: A Rural Health Clinic Experience

Heather D. Carter-Templeton, PhD, RN-BC[a],*, Lin Wu, MLIS, AHIP[b]

KEYWORDS

- Mobile technologies • iPads • Apps • Access to information
- Evidence-based nursing practice • Rural nurses • Nurses' perceptions

KEY POINTS

- Most rural nurses are in favor of using mobile devices to access evidence-based nursing (EBN) resources at the point of care despite the fact that they have limited use of electronic evidence-based information programs (EEIBP).
- Rural nurses had different interpretations of information literacy and evidence-based practice (EBP).
- Lack of time, experience, and training are the major barriers for rural nurses to learn how to use mobile devices to access EBN resources.
- Participants' information needs center on medication and diagnosis. When they have questions, they tend to turn to help from other nurses, electronic or print resources, or a combination of these.
- Past experience with mobile devices influences how enthusiastically nurses embrace EEIBP.

INTRODUCTION

EBP has become an expectation for nurses and health care providers to provide quality patient care. Nurses must access a great deal of information via electronic resources to stay well informed and up to date, yet little is known about how nurses in rural settings access and use evidence in their daily practice.[1] Although nurses must use evidence-based resources to provide evidence-based care, limited access

Funding for this project was provided by The University of Alabama Research Grants Committee (2012). Additional support was provided by The University of Alabama Office of Information Technology.

[a] Capstone College of Nursing, University of Alabama, 650 University Boulevard, Tuscaloosa, AL 35401, USA; [b] Medical Science Library, A&M University, Kingsville Campus, MSC 131, 1010 W, Avenue B, Kingsville, TX 78363, USA
* Corresponding author.
E-mail address: hcartertempleton@ua.edu

to evidence-based information is a barrier to research utilization in the clinical setting, especially in remote locations. his qualitative descriptive study determines the feasibility and usability of a mobile device to support clinical decision making in a rural health clinic via increasing access to and use of evidence-based information.

Mobile devices used in clinical settings include tablet computers, handheld computers, smartphones, and personal digital assistants (PDAs). Many reliable and credible evidence-based electronic repositories are available for download to mobile devices, providing quick access to valuable nursing information. Nurses who are proficient using mobile devices outfitted with these resources can gain access rapidly and as a result may bestow more suitable and efficient care to their clients.

STUDY AIM

The specific aim of this study was to describe the feasibility and usability of a mobile device and selected EEIBP used to support clinical decision making in a rural health clinic. This study focused on the nurses' descriptions of their experience with the selected mobile device and EEIBP.

LITERATURE REVIEW

Literature searches were conducted in the following databases: PubMed/Medline, CINAHL Plus with Full Text, Scopus, Web of Science, and Google Scholar. Search concepts included access to information, in-service training, EBN practice, mobile technologies, and rural or remote clinics or hospitals. The searches were limited to English language and the publication years from 2003 through October 2014.

Mobile technologies have opened new doors for nurses to access an array of online evidence-based resources, offered a solution for getting evidence to nurses directly at the point of care,[2] and connected learning and evidence to clinical care.[3] The study published by Doran and colleagues[4] in 2012 implies handheld portable devices support nurses' use of information resources in clinical practice.

Nurses who use PDAs believe that these devices support clinical decision making, promote patient safety, and increase productivity.[5] Using mobile devices can also promote timely communication, enabling evidence-based collaborative practice and supporting workplace learning.[6] Nurses who access resources using mobile devices are more efficient in determining an answer to the clinical questions.[7]

However, most nurses do not have adequate information technology and information literacy competencies[8,9] to access and use needed evidence-based information. In addition, nurses receive less education pertaining to information technology and information literacy than do most health care workers.[10] Gosling and colleagues[8] investigated the factors influencing nurses' use of the Web-based Clinical Information Access Program that provided online access to evidence-based resources at the point of care. They discovered that the most frequent reasons for not using the resources are lack of training and time; this is especially true for nurses who work at rural or remote health care facilities. A 2012 survey by the Healthcare Information Management System Society reveals that mobile technologies improved access to patient information and clinical information from remote locations[11] where access to information is often more limited and challenging.[12]

However, there is a lack of published literature concerning education received by nurses working in rural settings pertaining to the use of tablet computers for accessing evidence-based resources. Moreover, little guidance exists for teaching nurses how to use mobile devices and applications within the clinical setting.

STUDY DESIGN

Because little is known about how nurses in rural settings use EEIBP, this study used a qualitative descriptive design. In an effort to illuminate the phenomenon being studied, participants were purposefully recruited from nurses providing direct patient care at a rural health care clinic in the southern region of the United States. Data collection was divided into 3 phases including 3 data collection points for each participant over the course of 6 to 8 months: baseline, formative, and summative interviews. The purpose of this study was to explore feasibility and usability of a mobile device equipped with EEIBP; therefore, participants were not mandated to use the iPads. Furthermore, to avoid HIPAA (Health Insurance Portability and Accountability Act of 1996) violations and maintain patient confidentiality, the mobile devices were not linked to any documentation or electronic health record (EHR) within the facility. Participants did not download or view any private patient information via the mobile devices. The mobile device was used to gain information about clinical questions. Participants were asked about the frequency and specifics about how they were using the devices throughout the formative and summative interviews. Again, the use of the device was not mandated.

Potential participants were recruited through informational fliers about the study and through brief informational sessions at scheduled staff meetings. Inclusion criteria for the study included being employed at the study site as a licensed practical nurse or nurse practitioner.

Each participant received a 1-hour training program delivered by the principal investigator (PI) and a health science librarian after the baseline interview and on receiving their assigned iPad. The educational intervention was a 1-hour training session. The content used to educate the participants was the result of collaboration between a nursing faculty member and a health science librarian. FaceTime was used to connect the librarian into the training session with the PI and participants. During the session, the participants were instructed on iPad navigation basics, Skyscape software, and updating the iPad.

Participants were allowed to actively demonstrate skills as the content was shared, creating an awareness of the usefulness of mobile devices through demonstration of their applicability to actual clinical settings. The participants were also informed about the supplemental information from Skyscape vendor explaining searching basics for the application. In addition, content from an iPad2 starter guide that had been preloaded onto their assigned iPad was discussed. The starter guide contained basic information about the iPad, including information on settings, camera use, charging, updating, and syncing the device. These materials were loaded onto each iPad and could be used by participants if needed for future reference.

Audiotape-recorded interviews were conducted at 3 different points during the study. A standardized open-ended interview format with follow-up and probing questions was used to assist the researcher in the interviews. The interview guide included questions about times in which participants needed more information, where they sought information, what made them feel comfortable about the information they found, and rules and guidelines they used to determine if information should be used in patient care. This guide ensured standardization of questioning and helped the PI collect common information from each participant. In addition, a demographic questionnaire was used to collect data on age, gender, years licensed as a registered nurse, and educational history.

DATA COLLECTION AND ANALYSIS

Before data collection, the researcher obtained approval to proceed with the study from the Institutional Review Board at the university affiliated with the study site. All participants were offered an explanation of the study purpose and information about the expectations of being a participant in the study. Informed consent was obtained by each participant at each interview. Demographic information was collected from each participant during the baseline interview.

The primary data collection strategy was audio-recorded interviews with participants. A semistructured interview guide was used to systematically ask questions of participants. Audio files were transcribed verbatim into word processor files. Each participant interview was stored in separate files. File names included the data collection phase and a participant number. All transcripts were read to confirm completeness. The audio files were replayed while the transcript was read to verify accuracy of the content. Reading the transcripts multiple times facilitated familiarity with the data and assisted with data analysis.

Data analysis attempted to discover concepts and relationships from the raw data. Data were analyzed in 4 primary phases: (1) coding of raw deidentified data through first and second cycle coding, (2) codes were grouped into themes then compared among transcripts, (3) themes were analyzed and compared with other themes, and (4) concepts were summarized and conclusions about the data were made.[13] ATLAS.ti qualitative software was used to assist in data management throughout the study.

Data from transcripts were coded inductively and frequently based on emic examples offered by participants represented in the data. Analysis was first done by looking at responses to questions in each interview, then among all responses in each phase. Codes were developed based on responses to questions. An open coding technique was used as data were read and studied for relevance to the interview questions. This preliminary list of codes was used to code subsequent transcripts, often being edited to reflect new insight from new data. Second-level coding resulted in identifying new codes or editing existing ones and exploring commonalities and differences among interview data.

Codes across interviews were then grouped into themes. Descriptive statistics were used to summarize participants' demographic characteristics. These data were used to compare and contrast demographic information among participants. Themes were analyzed for patterns. Lastly, themes were categorized to develop conclusions.[13] A summary of the data analysis was offered to participants at the conclusion of the study. Participants agreed with the findings.

SETTINGS AND SAMPLE

The host site was a rural federally qualified health care center in western Alabama, providing care to approximately 2170 unique patients with 6300 total medical encounters per year. The facility had a reliable information technology infrastructure with Wi-Fi access and multiple desktop computers for nursing staff to use.

Participants (n = 7) represented a purposeful sample of 7 nurses (3 Licensed Practical Nurses [LPNs] and 4 Nurse Practitioners [NPs]) working in a rural health clinic. Of the 7 participants, 1 (14%) was a man and 6 (86%) were women. The average age of participants was 39 (range, 31–46) years, and they had been in the nursing profession for an average of 13 (range, 3–21) years. Participants had been at the clinic for an average of 4 (range, 1–10) years.

FINDINGS

The findings of this study were based on analysis of participants' responses to the interview questions in the baseline, formative, and summative interviews. The analysis process led to the identification the following themes: (1) information needs (2) different interpretations of EBP, (3) benefits and challenges of using mobile devices in the clinical setting. These themes along with additional findings are explained and illustrated with select excerpts from the interviews.

The results are reported in summary based on answers to the interview questions presented to participants.

Clinical Question Inquiry and Types of Information Needed

The process of information seeking and appraisal begins with a question or a prompt to seek additional information and ends once they receive information from the resource they trust. Variations in resources used were contingent on the type of clinical question, the urgency of the situation, resource accessibility, and/or credibility or reliability of resources. In many cases, participants described evaluating the resource of information, not necessarily the content provided by the resource. In addition, participants frequently discussed having discussions with other nurses when they explored their clinical questions. Participants reported using several applications to assist in the process of finding answers to their clinical questions including Skyscape, Epocrates, Google, and their calculator.

Types of Information Needs

Two types of information needs were predominately discussed among the participants: medication-related questions and questions about unfamiliar diagnoses.

Medication-related questions

Medication questions may be answered by other nurses, print or electronic resources, or a combination of these. Several participants commented that they turn to other nurses to collect baseline or cursory information about a drug and then pursued additional evidence-based information in hard or electronic format. Participants discussed evaluating electronic resources by past experience and comfort with the program or system. Print resources, such as drug books, were evaluated based on currency and were often used if they had been designated books or resources used while in nursing school.

Unfamiliar diagnosis–related questions

For diagnosis-related questions, participants reported using human, electronic, and/or print resources for additional information. Among the LPNs, the nurse practitioners were the most commonly named resource because of their role and knowledge. If LPNs or NPs were describing the use of an electronic resource, the evaluation was based on past experience with the program or system, if it was a reputable site, and if the information was being validated by several Web sites. If print resources were used, it was often based on availability or access.

Describing Evidence-Based Practice

Although there were variations in participants' exact descriptions of what they thought when they heard the term evidence-based practice, some participants were confident in their descriptions. Some described EBP as "showing and proving, shown and proved, that this is an effective treatment or, um, effective way to do, um, whatever procedure or whatever, um, tests, whatever you're doing in your nursing career." There were some who admitted confusion or not knowing what it really is. Another stated "really don't" know what EBP is, validating the need for continued education regarding EBP in the clinical setting.

Benefits and Challenges of Mobile Devices

Throughout the formative and summative interviews, participants were asked to describe if and how they were incorporating the mobile device into their day-to-day practices. During this portion of the interview, benefits of the device were often discussed. The most frequently cited benefits included use for patient teaching, ease of use when searching, and portability.

Throughout the study, participants frequently discussed how they were integrating the iPad into their day-to-day practices. A commonly cited use of the iPad was for patient teaching. Many participants remarked about the vivid images that assisted them in speaking with patients about disease processes or physical changes. One stated:

Because that really hits home to them when I'm doing counseling to a teenager who like maybe started birth control or something like that...I can talk about STDs and pull up pictures and say 'here you go.'

Another said:

And the fact that I can pull up pictures or something really fast and actually show it to the patient, that's a plus.

One said:

...I love that I can go and take it and show things to patients and the parents on the iPad in the room. Its very easy... they can see it a whole lot clearer versus just a printed picture from me sitting at a desktop and printing off... or something...they can see it right there in front of them.

Other participants discussed the easy and swift searching that can be done using a mobile device equipped with EEIBP. One participant stated:

...it has a main search tool that you just type in something and it pulls up everything it has on that.

Another participant said:

...just easy and fast to look up versus having to go look up a big drug guide where you have to hunt for everything.

One stated:

You don't have turn pages, its just right there.

Another benefit frequently noted was that of portability and size. Some commented that they were not bound to a desk with it. Specifically they stated:

...it's handy, I don't have to be sitting there at the desk I can just use it and walk off with it.

Another said:

...it's small...you can take it with you, you can take in the room and let them look at it. You know if it's a picture example or read the definition if it's something needs to be explained.

And probably most importantly were the comments related to the confidence it gave them. Some noted:

I think it gives you more confidence in the knowledge that you're passing along to the patient...for reassurance.

Although most participants described their experiences with the mobile devices and EEIBP as positive, some did offer insights into the challenges associated with using the devices in the clinical setting. Of the challenges discussed, cost was the most frequently cited. One stated:

…I don't have it because it's a paid app, it's like an expensive paid app…

Another said:

…I just don't have the app because I have the hard back book and it's so expensive to buy the app.

Another challenge noted by some participants in this study was the lack of a connected printer. Although it is possible to connect mobile devices to printers, it was not done with this study.
One said:

It would probably be more helpful if I was able to hook up to a printer and print things out for patients.

Another person said:

One thing that I can't do on it that I have to go my computer for is print. And so if like I want print a picture or something like that then I have to pull it up on my computer.

In addition to the above-mentioned challenges, several noted the benefit that would likely result from required electronic connections such as health records and documentation being accessible from the mobile device. One of the participants stated:

Your optimal situation would be to have these resources on the same platform, device…along with your EHR.

Planning learning experiences with mobile devices

Most of the participants had not taken a dedicated computer course as a nursing student or as a professional nurse. Most of any training related to technology had been provided to them onsite or it was related to the EHR system used at the clinics. Participants expressed preferences for how they would like to learn about new technology, such as the use of a mobile device, in the clinical setting. They specifically described the wish for more information on how to use specific applications, yet would also indicate that a lack of time could potentially keep them from participating in learning experiences.
Some described learning independently and gaining hands-on experience:

…you could stand there and talk to me all day long; it's not going to help. If I don't actually get it out and, you know, search on it and do it myself, so you have done as much as you can do for me.

Another person said:

…then I think for the most part they have to get their hands on it and you know…have some…just like how we do in class—give them some sort of assignment that makes them navigate through it and all the different resources that are available on that.

Past experience with mobile devices seemed to influence how enthusiastically EEIBP were embraced. Some discussed the advantage of being an experienced user of mobile devices:

…I've been able to, you know, move pretty freely through…easily. It was second nature to me.

IMPLICATIONS

Overall, the benefits for nurses using mobile devices in the rural clinical setting out-weighed the challenges associated with it. It was evident that each nurse may have chosen several ways to gain answers to those clinical questions they elected to explore. Decisions about what resources they used were contingent on several variables, including the urgency of the situation, the type of question, the availability of other nurses, and their familiarity with and availability of specific evidence-based resources.

Nurses proficient using mobile devices furnished with evidence-based resources can access important information quickly. Access to evidence-based information at the point of care is often necessary for nurses to apply up-to-date approaches in to-day's information-rich clinical settings. Lack of training and experience with technology can be a barrier to its use. Developing a teaching plan for educating the nurses on how to use mobile devices may assist in conveying information that may not be clearly understood by the user. The process of sharing helper information about the mobile device and evidence-based applications may be of assistance to the end user and can have an impact on the uptake and use of technology in the clinical setting.

Although access to Internet and evidence-based resources may exist for some nurses practicing in rural settings, the lack of skills regarding the interpretation of research and inconsistencies related to the value of research have been reported in the literature. Findings from this study provide helpful insight regarding the role of EEIBP in rural clinical nursing practice. Although most participants found it beneficial to incorporate the use of a mobile device equipped with evidence-based resources, they perceived that nurses other than themselves demonstrated limited use of EEIBP via mobile devices.

FUTURE RESEARCH

The results of this study provide a foundation for future research related to the development and use mobile devices in the rural clinical setting and training regarding mobile device applications. Yet the use of mobile devices in the rural clinical setting needs further research. More must be understood about the usability of information presented via mobile applications. Based on the results of this study, research related to the involvement of end users in the application development process is needed. In addition, research on the integration of the EHR within a mobile device platform needs to be explored. Finally, the use of more objective measures such as surveys and questionnaires would benefit this body of knowledge.

REFERENCES

1. O'Lynn C, Luparell S, Winters C, et al. Rural nurses' research use. Online J Rural Nurs Health Care 2009;9(1):34–45.
2. Doran DM, Haynes RB, Kushniruk A, et al. Supporting evidence-based practice for nurses through information technologies. Worldviews Evid Based Nurs 2010; 7(1):4–15.
3. Wyatt TH, Krauskopf PB, Gaylord NM, et al. Cooperative m-learning with nurse practitioner students. Nurs Educ Perspect 2010;31(2):109–13.
4. Doran D, Haynes BR, Estabrooks CA, et al. The role of organizational context and individual nurse characteristics in explaining variation in use of information technologies in evidence based practice. Implement Sci 2012;7:122.

5. Stroud SD, Smith CA, Erkel EA. Personal digital assistant use by nurse practitioners: a descriptive study. J Am Acad Nurse Pract 2009;21(1):31–8.
6. Doran DM. The emerging role of PDAs in information use and clinical decision making. Evid Based Nurs 2009;12(2):35–8.
7. Krauskopf PB, Farrell S. Accuracy and efficiency of novice nurse practitioners using personal digital assistants. J Nurs Scholarsh 2011;43(2):117–24.
8. Gosling AS, Westbrook JI, Spencer R. Nurses' use of online clinical evidence. J Adv Nurs 2004;47(2):201–11.
9. Winters CA, Lee HJ, Besel J, et al. Access to and use of research by rural nurses. Rural Remote Health 2007;7(3):758.
10. Alpay L, Russell A. Information technology training in primary care: the nurses' voice. Comput Inform Nurs 2002;20(4):136–42.
11. Boone E, Horowitz J. Show me the research - HIMSS mobile technology survey. 2012. Available at: http://www.himss.org/News/NewsDetail.aspx?ItemNumber=4722. Accessed December 15, 2014.
12. Anderson C, Henner T, Burkey J. Tablet computers in support of rural and frontier clinical practice. Int J Med Inf 2013;82(11):1046–58.
13. Miles MB, Huberman AM, Saldana J. Qualitative data analysis: a methods sourcebook. Los Angeles (CA): Sage Publications, Inc; 2014.

A Clinical Protocol for the Assessment of Obesity

Addressing an Epidemic

Candy S. Rinehart, DNP, FNP, ADM-BC[a],*, JoAnn S. Oliver, PhD, RN, CNE[b]

KEYWORDS

- Obesity • Obesity assessment • Weight loss • Educational interventions

KEY POINTS

- Obesity is underrecognized and undertreated in the primary care setting.
- Assessment of obesity is important in addressing the obesity epidemic.
- A clinical protocol could aid in initiating a conversation about weight.

PROBLEM

There are multiple sources of data available that describe the prevalence of obesity in the United States. The statistics from the Centers for Disease Control and Prevention (2012),[1] report that 69.2% of adults aged 20 years and older are overweight, including 35.9% who are obese. Similarly, in a study published in the *Journal of the American Medical Association*, researchers evaluating the 2011 to 2012 National Health and Nutrition Examination Survey data found that 34.9% of adults in this same age group were obese.[2] During their annual meeting in June 2013, the American Medical Association (AMA)[3] passed a policy that defined obesity as a disease. This policy identified the need for obesity treatment and prevention to improve health outcomes. Furthermore, supporters of the policy expressed hope that by defining obesity as a disease there would be more focus on the epidemic and more responsibility assumed on the part of health insurers. Additionally, the Affordable Care Act identifies obesity as a substantial health threat and provides coverage, without cost sharing, for obesity screening and counseling on healthy eating and weight loss to better address the increasing epidemic.

The body mass index (BMI) is the most widely used tool for the assessment of obesity. The BMI is calculated from the measured weight and height of a person and correlates with the amount of body fat. BMI is not to be interpreted as a direct

Disclosures: none.
[a] The Ohio State University College of Nursing, 1585 Neil Avenue, Columbus, OH 43210, USA;
[b] The University of Alabama, Capstone College of Nursing, 650 University Boulevard East, Tuscaloosa, AL 35401, USA
* Corresponding author.
E-mail address: rinehart.215@osu.edu

http://dx.doi.org/10.1016/j.cnur.2015.05.013
0029-6465/15/$ – see front matter © 2015 Elsevier Inc. All rights reserved.
nursing.theclinics.com

measure of body fat. An adult is defined as obese if the BMI is 30 or higher. A person with a healthy weight has a BMI range of 18.5 to 24.9. Individual BMI within the range of 25.0 to 29.9 is assessed as overweight.[4]

The health and economic consequences of obesity include direct and indirect medical costs that significantly impact the US health care system. The health consequences of obesity are numerous and include the risk and consequences of cardiovascular disease, type 2 diabetes, hypertension, cerebrovascular disease, dyslipidemia, and osteoarthritis.[5] Various types of cancer, gallstones, and disability are also included in the associated comorbid conditions. All of these consequences are associated with a higher use of health care services and higher costs for the person with obesity.[6] The medical care costs of obesity in the United States in 2008 are reported to have totaled the staggering amount of about $147 billion.[1] The Agency for Healthcare Research and Quality[5] reported that 72 million Americans are obese and more likely to suffer with chronic health problems.

GUIDELINES AND SUPPORT FOR PRACTICE CHANGE

Established guidelines, recommendations, and requirements for screening adults for obesity and obesity risks and providing weight loss interventions for overweight/obese adults are available from multiple organizations. The Healthcare Effectiveness Data and Information Set guidelines recommend that adults between 18 and 74 years of age receive BMI assessment annually at their primary care office visits.[7] The U S Preventive Services Task Force (USPSTF) recommends screening of all adults for obesity. The USPSTF recommendation applies to adults aged 18 years and older. Patients with a BMI of 30 or greater should immediately be offered or referred for counseling and behavioral interventions to promote weight loss.[5] The 2006 guidelines from the National Institute for Health and Clinical Excellence (NICE)[8] recommend that all primary care settings ensure that there are systems in place to provide interventions to prevent and manage obesity among children and adults. This NICE clinical guideline further promotes interventions to increase physical activity and improve diet. Evidence-based initiatives that include guideline integration offer the potential to improve the patient's outcomes, the quality of care provided to patients with obesity, and may prevent obesity in individuals who are overweight or at risk for the disease.[9,10]

BARRIERS AND BENEFITS

Application of guidelines should begin with routinely assessing patients for obesity as the initial step in addressing barriers to obesity management.[11] A review of the literature revealed that primary care professionals underrecognize and undertreat obesity. In a cross-sectional study by Melamed and colleagues[12] (2009), family practice physicians in 7 family practices documented BMI on only 35.3% of the patients. The study also found that only 12.8% of the medical records of obese patients that did not have a BMI documented also included an appropriate obesity diagnosis. This less-than-optimal rate of obesity assessment correlated with the low rate of obesity interventions and weight-loss counseling. Bardia and colleagues[13] (2007) used a primary care database to review 9827 patient visits in a primary care clinic. It was found that 19.9% of the 2542 patients with obesity had a documented diagnosis of obesity. Identified as a benefit, the presence of documentation substantiating an obesity diagnosis correlated with an increased chance of an obesity management plan also being formulated and documented.

In addition to the lack of BMI documentation and appropriate inclusion of the obesity diagnosis in the medical record, there are practice barriers that have been identified that prevent the primary care provider (PCP) from advising and motivating patients about weight loss.[14–17] Day-to-day factors identified as key barriers to obesity assessment and interventions include the skill and knowledge of the PCP, inconsistent obesity management guidelines, resource availability, and the provider's personal attitudes and beliefs about obesity.[17,18] Additional barriers for the PCP to managing obesity and individuals at risk for obesity include lack of time, limited referral options, seeming lack of success with previous interventions and high rates of relapse, and the perceived psychological complexity of obesity interventions.[16] Limited practitioner skills and confidence, lack of consistency of care, and general denial of the responsibility for obesity management were identified as barriers by Gunther and colleagues[15] (2012) in a qualitative study that looked at barriers to implement the NICE guidelines for the management of overweight and obese individuals. In summary, there is an identified need for simple and effective interventions, in the primary care setting, for individuals who are obese or at risk for obesity.[19,20] The success of obesity interventions depend on the approach taken and the support that is provided.[14]

The benefits and harms of obesity assessment and interventions are reviewed in the recommendations by the USPSTF.[6] Weight decrease was a benefit described by the USPSTF when using intensive multicomponent behavioral interventions. Contrary to this, the USPSTF also identified potential harms. Decreased bone mineral density, increased fracture, serious injuries resulting from increased physical activities, and increased risk of eating disorders were some of the potential harms described in the final USPSTF recommendation statement.[6] According to Moyer[21] (2012), included in the clinical summary of these recommendations is evidence that the harms of screening for obesity and providing behavioral interventions are small. The USPSTF further concluded that there is a moderate net benefit in obesity screening.[6] LeBlanc and colleagues[22] (2011) also reviewed the harms and effectiveness of primary care–based obesity interventions and reported that behavioral weight-loss interventions did produce clinically meaningful weight loss.

OBESITY AND ASSESSMENT

In a review of primary care physicians' recognition and management of obesity, Fujioka and Bakhru[23] (2010) ask, "How do we treat the disease if [it] is not diagnosed?"[23(pp 467)] Therefore, how do patients know that they are obese or at risk for obesity if it has not been assessed? The collection of quantitative data is included in the assessment and problem-solving phases of the nursing process.[24] Measuring height and weight is the initial quantitative data necessary to calculate the BMI (via the electronic health record [EHR] or a calculating tool). Also relevant is educating patients about BMI definitions, the need for an assessment of weight, and any risk factors for being overweight or obese.

Integrating the BMI as a vital sign is a powerful tool that leads to the first step in recognizing and improving obesity interventions.[23] Measuring height and weight to attain the BMI allows for the opportunity to begin discussions regarding weight loss, risk reduction, and lifestyle changes.[25] Assessing for obesity and obesity risk in this clinical protocol begins with the support staff attaining BMI information along with the other vital signs collected for the primary care visit (ie, blood pressure, pulse, and respiratory rate). These data are then included in the patients' medical record. Saviñon and colleagues[26] (2012) noted that, in their study, BMI documentation improved 62% because of structured staff training and the electronic medical record.

SUPPORT FOR LIFESTYLE MODIFICATION

Koh and Sebelius (2010)[27] discuss the Affordable Care Act and the prevention themes that are highlighted. The Affordable Care Act addresses obesity as a substantial health threat and includes coverage, with no cost sharing, for obesity screening and counseling for adults and children. This initiative further supports the utilization of a clinical protocol within the clinical setting. A clinical protocol provides guidance and a framework for consistent overweight and obesity screening and providing education and counseling focused on lifestyle modification to prevent or treat obesity.

Kirk and colleagues[28] (2012) support the use of evidence-based guidelines that promote lifestyle interventions for the individual with obesity. Current treatment options for those that are obese or at risk for obesity include promotion of weight loss through lifestyle interventions and behavior modification. Even modest weight loss accompanied by physical activity has been shown to reduce obesity-related coronary heart disease risk factors.[29] Furthermore, the evidence suggests that multicomponent interventions that include behavioral change, dietary counseling, and physical activity are likely to be the most effective.[20,28,30]

There is a recognized need in the primary care setting for a standardized, multicomponent, easily understood lifestyle intervention that could be provided once patients are assessed as obese or at risk for obesity. Included in the practice protocol is information from the (AHA).[31] The AHA[31] was used as a source to develop a handout for patients identified as obese or at risk for obesity and in need of lifestyle interventions. The "5 Goals to Losing Weight" strategies consist of multicomponent interventions that contain lifestyle-modification activities that monitor portion sizes, encourage low-caloric food choices, suggest tracking food intake, support reducing or eliminating foods high in fat and sugar, and include incorporating physical activity. The written information includes materials specific for patients regarding BMI and the "5 Goals to Losing Weight" in a single-page handout format.[31]

DESCRIPTION OF THE CLINICAL PRACTICE PROTOCOL

The practice protocol for the primary care setting begins with the medical assistants (MAs) attaining and recording an accurate height, weight, and BMI within the EHR at every patient visit. The BMI is automatically calculated when height and weight measurements are entered (height can be carried forward).

All patients with a BMI greater than 30 will have a documented diagnosis of obesity in the Today's Assessments area of the EHR, which will automatically enter this diagnosis into the diagnosis history of the health record. All patients with a BMI greater than 25 will be provided with a written handout that defines BMI by healthy, overweight, obese, or morbidly obese (**Box 1**). This handout will also include documentation of patients' present BMI.

Finally, the clinical protocol will include a standardized behavioral intervention for lifestyle modification to be provided in a written format to all patients with BMIs equal to or greater than 25. This handout will include the "5 Goals to Losing Weight."[31] This behavioral intervention provides day-to-day strategies for food and activity with the goal of using more calories than are consumed. The information is presented in easy-to-understand concepts and format and can be readily viewed and shared on the AHA's Web site:

1. Keep portions smaller than your fist.
2. Control your hunger with filling foods that are low in calories.
3. Keep track of what you eat.
4. Make trade-offs to reduce how much fat and sugar you eat.
5. Enjoy more physical activity

Box 1
BMI and weight loss information

Weight Classification	BMI (kg/m^2)
Underweight	<18.5
Normal	18.5–24.9
Overweight	25.0–29.9
Obesity: class 1	30.0–34.9
Obesity: class 2	35.0–39.9
Extreme obesity	$\geq$40.0

Patient name: _____

Date: _____

BMI: _____

"5 Goals to Losing Weight" (AHA/Learn and Live)

Includes strategies for food and physical activity:

1. Keep portion smaller than your fist. This practice helps with overeating. A reasonable portion size for most food is 0.5 to 1.0 cup. Exceptions to this rule would be that portions of meat, chicken, and fish should be the size of a deck of cards (which is smaller than your fist) and eating as much plain vegetables and salad (these foods are low in calories and are filling).

2. Control your hunger with filling foods that are low in calories. Salad, fruits, soups, and vegetables help you lose weight by satisfying hunger.

3. Keep track of what you eat. Keep a food log or diary.

4. Make trade-offs to reduce how much fat and sugar you eat. Eat a smaller meal if you are going to have dessert.

5. Enjoy more physical activity: a total of 150 minutes of moderate-intensity physical activity per week.

Additional information is available from the AHA's Web site: http://www.heart.org/HEARTORG/GettingHealthy/WeightManagement/LosingWeight/5-Goals-to-Losing-Weight_UCM_307260_Article.jsp.

Data from National Heart, Lung, and Blood Institute. The practical guide: identification, evaluation, and treatment of overweight and obesity in adults. 2000. Available at: http://www.nhlbi.nih.gov/guidelines/obesity/ob_gdlns.pdf.

Additional documentation in the EHR will reflect the behavioral intervention and the patients' questions or responses to the intervention.

The integration of a practice protocol for obesity requires a team effort among the disciplines within the primary care practice. The MAs are responsible for obtaining and documenting height, weight, and BMI in the EHR. The MAs and the clerical staff will need to ensure that the handouts are available for each patient intervention. The nurse practitioner providers will be responsible for consistently following the clinical protocol and address any barriers to adherence and patient or staff concerns or make suggestions for ongoing improvement to the clinical protocol.

SUMMARY

The health and economic consequences of obesity significantly impact the US health care system.[1,5] Although the AMA passed a policy that defines obesity as a disease, the review of the literature revealed a low rate of assessment and documentation of the diagnosis of obesity in the primary care setting. The rapidly increasing incidence of obesity, which severely impacts health and economics, and the insufficient amount of diagnosis support the need for evidence-based clinical practice protocols to assess for obesity and obesity risks within our primary care population.

Translation of evidence-based guidelines into a new clinical protocol for the primary care setting uses the nursing process. Initially, identifying the need to assess for obesity and obesity risks with BMI data provides an excellent foundation to identifying the problem. The important documentation of BMI data and an obesity diagnosis when appropriate further provides support to help patients and the PCP start a conversation about weight issues with objective data to support a need for change. These steps are important when making a shared decision on integrating a plan for weight-management strategies into an intervention. Multiple behavioral interventions are needed to address the obesity epidemic. Implementation of a clinical protocol focused on the assessment of obesity may be an important first step.

REFERENCES

1. Centers for Disease Control and Prevention. Adult obesity facts. 2012. Available at: http://www.cdc.gov/nchs/data/databriefs/db82.pdf. Accessed February 24, 2013.
2. Ogden CL, Carroll MD, Kit BK, et al. Prevalence of childhood and adult obesity in the United State, 2011-2012. J Am Med Assoc 2014;11(8):806–14.
3. AMA defines obesity as a disease. Clinical advisor. Available at: http://www.clinicaladvisor.com/ama-defines-obesity-as-a-disease/article/299775/?DCMP=EMC-CA_UPDATE&cpn=ca_cympn;450&spMailingID=6431215&spUserID=MTM2Nzc1NzQ4ODMS1&spJobID=76749028&spReportId=NzY3NDkwMjgS1. Accessed June 21, 2013.
4. National Heart, Lung and Blood Institute. The practical guide: identification, evaluation, and treatment of overweight and obesity in adults. 2000. Available at: http://www.nhlbi.nih.gov/guidelines/obesity/ob_gdlns.pdf. Accessed March 15, 2013.
5. Agency for Healthcare Research and Quality. National healthcare disparities report. AHRQ publication No. 13–0003. 2012. Available at: http://www.ahrq.gov/research/findings/nhqrdr/nhdr12/2012nhdr.pdf. Accessed February 14, 2013.
6. U.S. Preventive Services Task Force. Screening for and management of obesity in adults: clinical summary of U.S. Preventive Services Task Force recommendation. AHRQ publication No. 11-05149EF-3. 2012. Available at: http://www.uspreventiveservicestaskforce.org/uspstf11/obeseadult//obesesum.htm. Accessed March 16, 2013.
7. National Committee for Quality Assurance. The state of health care quality 2012. 2012. Available at: http://wwwncqa.org/Portals/0/State%20of%20Health%20Care/2012/SOHC%20Report%20Web.pdf. Accessed March 16, 2013.
8. National Institute for Health and Clinical Excellence. Obesity guidance on the prevention, identification, assessment and management of overweight and obesity in adults and children. 2006. Available at: http://www.nice.org.uk/nicemedia/live/11000/30365030365.pdf. Accessed February 14, 2013.
9. Farrah N, Ellis P, Barron ML. Assessment of provider adherence to obesity treatment guidelines. J Am Assoc Nurse Pract 2013;25(3):147–55.
10. Melnyk BM, Fineout-Overholt E. Evidence-based practice in nursing and healthcare: a guide to best practice. Philadelphia: Lippincott Williams & Wilkins; 2011.
11. Turner M, Burns SM, Knight L, et al. Weight management practices among heart and vascular health care providers in an ambulatory setting. Medsurg Nurs 2012; 21(4):222–32.

12. Melamed OC, Nakar S, Vinker S. Suboptimal identification of obesity by family physicians. Am J Manag Care 2009;15(9):619–24.

13. Bardia A, Holtan SG, Slezak JM, et al. Diagnosis of obesity by primary care physicians and impact on obesity management. Mayo Clin Proc 2007;82(8):927–32.

14. Hindle L, Mills S. Obesity: self-care and illness prevention. Pract Nurs 2012;13(3): 130–4.

15. Gunther S, Guo F, Sinfield P, et al. Barriers and enablers to managing obesity in general practice: a practical approach for use in implementation activities. Qual Prim Care 2012;20(2):93–103.

16. Nolan C, Deehan A, Jones R. Practice nurses and obesity: professional and practice-based factors affecting role adequacy and role legitimacy. Prim Health Care Res Dev 2012;13:353–63.

17. Walsh MAF, Fahy KM. Interaction between primary health care professionals and people who are overweight or obese: a critical review. Aust J Adv Nurs 2011; 29(2):23–9.

18. Hopkins K, DeCristofaro C, Elliot L. How can primary care providers manage pediatric obesity in the real world? J Am Acad Nurse Pract 2011;23:278–88.

19. Beeken RJ, Croker HH, Morris SS, et al. Study protocol for the 10 Top Tips (10TT) Trial: randomised controlled trial of habit-based advice for weight control in general practice. BMC Public Health 2012;667. http://dx.doi.org/10.1186/1471-2458-12-667.

20. Shay L, Shobert J, Seibert D, et al. Adult weight management: translating research and guidelines into practice. J Am Acad Nurse Pract 2009;21:197–206.

21. Moyer VA. Screening for and management of obesity in adults: U.S. Preventive Services Task Force recommendation statement. Ann Intern Med 2012;157(5):373–8.

22. LeBlanc E, O'Connor E, Whitlock E, et al. Effectiveness of primary care-relevant treatments for obesity in adults: a systematic review for the U.S. Preventive Services Task Force. Ann Intern Med 2011;155(7):434–47.

23. Fujioka K, Bakhru N. Office-based management of obesity. Mt Sinai J Med 2010; 77(5):466–71.

24. Broom M. Exploring the assessment process. Paediatr Nurs 2007;19(4):22–5.

25. Burke LE, Wang J. Treatment strategies for overweight and obesity. J Nurs Scholarsh 2011;43(4):368–75.

26. Saviñon C, Taylor JS, Canty-Mitchell J, et al. Childhood obesity: can electronic medical records customized with clinical practice guidelines improve screening and diagnosis? J Am Acad Nurse Pract 2012;24(8):463–71.

27. Koh HK, Sebelius KG. Promoting prevention through the Affordable Care Act. N Engl J Med 2010. http://dx.doi.org/10.1056/NEJMp1008560.

28. Kirk SF, Penney TL, McHugh TL, et al. Effective weight management practice: a review of the lifestyle intervention evidence. Int J Obes (Lond) 2012;36(2):178–85.

29. Klein S, Burke L, Bray G, et al. Clinical implications of obesity with specific focus on cardiovascular disease - a statement for professionals from the American Heart Association Council on Nutrition, Physical Activity, and Metabolism - endorsed by the American College of Cardiology Foundation. Circulation 2004; 110(18):2952–67.

30. Flodgren G. Interventions to change the behaviour of health professionals and the organisation of care to promote weight reduction in overweight and obese adults. Cochrane Database Syst Rev 2010;(12):CD000984.

31. American Heart Association. Getting healthy: 5 goals to losing weight. 2012. Available at: http://www.heart.org/HEARTORG/GettingHealthy/WeightManagement/LosingWeight/5-Goals-to-Losing-Weight_UCM_307260_Article.jsp#.UQXhCO0c27s. email.

Rural Health and the Nonemergency Use of Emergency Medical Services

 CrossMark

LaWanda W. Baskin, MSN, APRN, FNP-C[a],*,
Janelle R. Baker, PhD, APRN, A-GPCNP-BC[a],
Teresa L. Bryan, MSN, APRN, FNP-BC[b],
Geraldine Q. Young, DNP, FNP-BC[a],
Yolanda M. Powell-Young, PhD, PCNS-BC, CPN[c]

KEYWORDS

- Rural health • Emergency treatment • Health care reform • Access to health care
- Health care disparities

KEY POINTS

- Findings from this research suggest factors related to medical necessity were the most frequently cited for using ED services for non-emergent care.
- Socioeconomic status and type of insurance was less frequently cited as reasons for accessing the ED for non-emergent care.
- The respondents' perceived their condition warranted emergency treatment even though all participants were triaged at a non-emergent level.
- Findings from several research studies suggest that inadequate health literacy is a practical risk factor for inappropriate use of hospital ED services.

More than 50 million Americans living in rural areas are faced with challenges accessing health care.[1] Rural communities comprise 25% of the United States' population; however, less than 10% of primary care providers (PCPs) practice in rural communities.[2,3] It is estimated that there are only 65 primary care physicians per 100,000 rural Americans, which is 40 less than the 105 per 100,000 urban and suburban Americans. Thus, the shortage of PCPs in rural America has been influential in this vulnerable population's decision to seek care in Emergency Departments (EDs) for nonemergent

Funding Sources: None.
Conflicts of Interest: None.
[a] Graduate Nursing Programs, Alcorn State University, 15 Campus Drive, Natchez, MS 39120, USA; [b] FNP Track, Alcorn State University, 15 Campus Drive, Natchez, MS 39120, USA; [c] School of Nursing, Alcorn State University, 15 Campus Drive, Natchez, MS 39120, USA
* Corresponding author.
E-mail address: lbaskin@alcorn.edu

health conditions.[4] Grant and colleagues[5] explored this problem in a rural community in the Mississippi Delta, and results suggest that difficulties accessing PCPs were more likely in areas where there were health care provider shortages.

The ED has become an attractive alternative to primary care in rural communities.[5] According to Berry,[6] more than 50% of rural ED visits were classified nonemergent and more than 50% of these visits to the rural ED take place during daytime business hours (9 AM to 5 PM). The US rural utilization of the ED increases the total health care expenditures and amplifies these trends. It is estimated that the gross charges in rural EDs were more than 5 million dollars.[6] Therefore, the purpose of this descriptive cross-sectional study is to describe the factors that influence a rural person's decisions to seek care in the ED in rural southeastern United States.

METHODOLOGY
Research Design and Sample

This descriptive cross-sectional design was used to discover the contributing factors most frequently cited for nonemergent use of ED services among rural-dwelling individuals living in Concordia parish in Southeast Louisiana. Data collection occurred over a 4-week period between November 2011 and January 2012. Information was collected from a convenience sample of N = 59 adults 18 years of age and older. Inclusion criteria included willingness to complete the directed interview and medical acuity (per triage protocol) of level 4 (non-urgent) or level 5 (minor) priorities. Although clients less than the age of 18 years could not participate as research participants, their legal guardians who were at least 18 years of age were considered eligible for participation in the research study. Individuals who were unable to speak and understand English, those who were cognitively or medically impaired to a degree that would prohibit adequate interview response, and those who were referred to the ED department by a health care provider were excluded from study participation. Data collection occurred in designated areas that provided adequate privacy Monday through Friday from the hours of 0800 to 1700. This time frame is generally accepted as standard for primary care practice office operations.

Human Subjects Protection

Before the implementation of recruitment procedures, written approvals to conduct the study were obtained from the Alcorn State University Institutional Review Board and the Executive Board from the selected hospitals. As part of the agreement for inclusion, prospective participants (a) received verbal and written information about the study protocol; (b) were informed that study inclusion was voluntary and as such were free to withdraw from the study completely or to refuse to answer particular questions at any time; (c) were advised that all information would be presented in the aggregate; and (d) were told that a decision not to participate in the study would not impact their medical care. Verbal response to questions asked by the research interviewer denoted initial and continued consent for study involvement. Volunteers were not compensated for their participation.

Data Source

The Emergency Medicine Patients' Access to Healthcare (EMPATH) instrument was used to collect data on factors that may influence the nonemergent use of ED services. This instrument was developed and piloted at the Department of Emergency Medicine at Mount Sinai School of Medicine. Details regarding the development, use, and psychometric properties of the EMPATH instruments are published in detail elsewhere.[7]

Briefly, the instrument consisted of questions that solicited information in 4 domains: demographic, medical acuity, access to care, and reasons for seeking care in the ED. Birth date and self-reported ancestry comprised the demographic domain. Presenting complaint and symptom duration were used to determine each participant's level of medical acuity. Access to health care was determined with 5 items that focused on access to and use of non-ED health providers. The final domain consisted of 21 items whereby level of agreement measured on a 3-point Likert scale (strongly agree, agree, and disagree) were used to determine individual perceptions of why ED services were used for their current complaint. Primary psychometric validation was conducted with pilot data that were generated from a volunteer sample of 1008 adults recruited from 28 urban and suburban hospitals across the nation. Common factor analysis estimated single-item reliability with the current sample.[8] According to Harmon, as reported by Wanous and Hudy,[9(p363)] the reliable variance for an item is the sum of its communality and its specificity. Thus, communality can be considered a conservative estimate of single-item reliability. The reliability indices (r) generated for the 21 items that speak to reasons for coming to the ED ranged from 0.50 to 0.87 with the current sample.

Statistical Analyses

All data were entered into a computerized database. Coded data were analyzed using the SPSS. Before analyses, all variables were edited separately for accuracy, completion, credible values, and violation of statistical assumptions. Sample-wide medians were substituted for the missing values. Demographic characteristics and sample responses were summarized using counts (percentages) and central tendency measurement.

For the purposes of the analyses presented here, the 3-option categories regarding levels of agreement for the 21 items related to the current use of ED services were collapsed into 2 categories: agree (strongly agree + agree) and disagree. Several considerations guided the category adjustments. These considerations included the study's primary aim of determining what factor or factors motivated the use of ED services for nonemergent care. By consolidating the strongly agree + agree response options, the authors thought that the conceptual variance between the 2 responses would not substantively alter the performance of the instrument or interpretation integrity.[10]

χ^2 goodness of fit was used to test group differences in proportion by insurance group (ie, insured vs uninsured). Fisher's exact test was used when expected frequencies were less than 1 in any cell or less than 5 in more than 20% of the cells. Statistical significance was set at $P<.05$ and analyzed with a post-hoc Bonferroni to correct for multiple comparisons.

RESULTS
Sample Characteristics

Respondents ranged in ages from 18 through 91 years of age (Mean$_{age}$ = 43.5 ± 14.8 years). The sample cohort was comprised of African Americans (63%, n = 37) and European Americans (37%, n = 22). Approximately 42% of the study sample reported that Medicaid or Medicare as their primary source of health care insurance coverage. Thirty-six percent (n = 21) of the sample reported no health care insurance coverage. Private insurance coverage (11%), workman's compensation (7%), and other forms of coverage such as Veterans' benefits (4%) comprised the remaining 22% of information related to health care coverage. Less than one-quarter (20%) of the study participants sought treatment from a health care provider before accessing ED services.

Reasons for Nonemergent Use of Emergency Department Services

In general, factors related to medical necessity were the most frequently cited for using ED services for nonemergent care. Among individuals in this sample, convenience items seem to be the second most frequently cited for using ED department services for nonemergent conditions. Financial and affordability elements were less frequently cited as motivations for accessing the ED for nonemergent care. Access and affordability factors seemed to be some of the least important motivators for accessing the ED during standard operating hours (ie, 0800–1700). More than 60% of sample respondents consistently agreed that insurability and financial solvency were not major considerations when making decisions to use the ED for nonemergent use. **Table 1** provides an overview of frequency summaries by study respondents.

Differences for Nonemergent Use of Emergency Department Services by Insurability Groupings

This study found statistically significant differences by insurance groups for 5 of the 21 survey items relative to nonemergent use of ED services. Comparative responses indicated that insured respondents agreed more frequently that the ED was the right place

Table 1
Frequency summary comparisons for reasons given by sample respondents for using the Emergency Department for nonemergent conditions

Item	All Respondents N = 59 Agree % (n)	Uninsured Respondents n = 21 Agree % (n)	Insured Respondents n = 38 Agree % (n)
1. Too worried about my problem	97 (57)	91 (19)	100 (38)
2. ED is the right place for this problem	90 (53)	76 (16)	97 (37)
3. This is a medical emergency	85 (50)	81 (17)	87 (33)
4. I am too sick or injured to go elsewhere	85 (50)	86 (18)	84 (32)
5. I am in too much pain	85 (50)	91 (19)	82 (31)
6. ED is closest/easiest place	81 (48)	76 (16)	84 (32)
7. No appointment necessary	76 (45)	71 (15)	79 (30)
8. Everything can be done here	49 (29)	71 (15)	40 (15)
9. No place other than ED	48 (28)	57 (12)	42 (16)
10. Regular care at this hospital	41 (24)	81 (17)	18 (7)
11. I have no insurance	39 (23)	100 (21)	0
12. I cannot afford other places	36 (21)	95 (20)	3 (1)
13. My medical records here	32 (19)	43 (9)	26 (10)
14. Family/friend told me to come	19 (11)	10 (2)	26 (10)
15. I like environment in the ED	10 (6)	14 (3)	8 (3)
16. ED is only place open	3 (2)	0	5 (2)
17. Other places don't take my insurance	3 (2)	—	0
18. Better medical care here	3 (2)	0	5 (2)
19. I need my prescriptions refilled	3 (2)	5 (1)	3 (2)
20. Staff speaks my language	0	0	0
21. I don't like my regular care facility	0	0	0

Percentages rounded to reflect whole numbers.

to go for their current medical complaint, χ^2 (2, N = 59) = 6.64, P = .02. In contrast, uninsured respondents were more likely to agree that the ED was their most affordable option, χ^2 (2, N = 59) = 50.60, P = .000; everything that was needed to treat their current medical condition was available at the ED, χ^2 (2, N = 59) = 6.65, P = .04; the ED was where they routinely received health care services, χ^2 (2, N = 59) = 21.92, P = .000; and that having no insurance was a key reason for accessing the ED for non-emergent care, χ^2 (2, N = 59) = 51.03, P = .000.

DISCUSSION

Nationally, Americans are becoming increasingly reliant on the hospital ED for ambulatory care–sensitive conditions. Goals of the current health care reform system are to provide efficient, cost-effective care in the appropriate treatment setting. As such, identifying and understanding reasons that motivate individuals to seek care in hospital EDs for nonurgent use are critical to improving access to care and the overall health of the nation.

Factors that have been consistently identified in the literature as influencing ED overuse include a lack of access to timely primary care services, designation as a medically underserved area or population, financial and legal obligations by hospitals to evaluate all clients who arrive in the ED, sources of payment for health care, and immediate reassurance about their medical condition.[11–13] Much of the data used to support current determinations regarding inappropriate ED use have been gathered from individuals residing in urban and suburban areas. Little is known about factors that influence the inappropriate use of ED services among adult individuals living in rural locales.

When compared with the few studies that have evaluated factors influencing ED services for nonemergent use, findings from the authors' study revealed both similarities and differences. Medical necessity was substantiated as the most frequently cited reasons for visiting the ED for nonemergent treatment among individuals in the current study.[7,14] In addition, some items associated with convenience such as "ED proximity" and "no appointment requirements" were frequently identified by participants in this study as reasons for nonemergent use of hospital ED services. These findings are similar to those reported by Ragin and colleagues.[7] However, other items that denote convenience, such as "medical records are here" and "everything can be done in the ED," were not as frequently identified as principal reasons for visiting the ED for nonemergent treatment. These findings were similar to those reported in a systematic review conducted by Carret and colleagues[15] of published studies related to prevalence and associated factors of inappropriate use of emergency services.

Study findings indicated affordability as an important factor for nonemergent use of hospital ED services. As expected, this frequency pattern was observed at a greater proportion among the uninsured participants in this study. The use of the ED as the PCP of choice for uninsured participants in this study establishes a compelling link among insurance availability, insurance/health services affordability, and health care decision-making.

Ragin and colleagues[7] hypothesized a preference for the hospital ED as a PCP among their study sample. However, researchers in the current study consider the interrelatedness of preference items, such as "regular care," "medical records here," and "like the ED environment," as a practical connection of (affordability) necessity rather than a preference alternative.

A notable finding in this study was that the respondents' perceived that their condition warranted emergency treatment even though all participants were triaged at a nonemergent level. Findings from several research studies suggest that the role of low health literacy may be a practical risk factor for inappropriate use of hospital ED services.[16–18] Consideration for the development and implementation of tailored health literacy programs targeted to reduce the inappropriate use of ED services may be a step in the right direction toward promoting informed health and health care decisions.

Strengths and Limitations

A few limitations should be discussed regarding these study findings. The descriptive nature and nonprobability sampling make it difficult to generalize the results beyond this sample. The aging of the population make the elderly increased users of the ED department for reasons that may differ from those of younger or middle-aged adults. This finding does not mean, however, that the use of ED services is appropriate or that impact factors for the elder subgroup are equivalent to those identified by individuals from other age groups. The inclusion of educational level as a covariable would also allow researchers to determine whether education might explain the differences or lack of differences in outcome measures between the groups. Future researchers should aim to recruit larger, more representative samples of clearly distinct adult subgroups of both genders. Further studies are needed to investigate potential variability across the age continuum.

These limitations notwithstanding, results from this study contribute to advancing the body of research related to ED use for primary care services with vulnerable populations. At present, knowledge about motivators that influence nonemergent use of ED services is limited. Information is especially sparse for adults residing in rural locales. Although more research is needed, these findings provide much needed insight into individual and group perceptions of barriers and facilitators of health care utilization.

SUMMARY

To the authors' knowledge, this is one of the few studies to evaluate factors that influence the utilization of hospital ED services for nonurgent use among a subsample of the population that is often disparately affected by health burdens. Although more research is needed, results from this study have important implications for health care utilization. Overall, the findings provide clearly needed insight regarding population-specific reasons adult clients living in the rural United States seek care in hospital EDs. Understanding the context of health and illness among vulnerable populations can inform the development and implementation of effective prevention and intervention strategies that address health disparities and inequities.

REFERENCES

1. U.S. Census Bureau. American Community Survey. 2009.
2. Ginde AA, Sullivan AF, Camargo CA Jr. National study of the emergency physician workforce, 2008. Ann Emerg Med 2009;54:349–59.
3. Hines A, Fraze T, Stocks C. Healthcare Cost and Utilization Project (HCUP) statistical briefs. Rockville (MD): New England Healthcare Institute; 2006.
4. Young D. Lack of primary care, insurance lead to urgent conditions: emergency care visits highest for blacks, uninsured. Am J Health Syst Pharm 2007;64: 1674–6.
5. Grant R, Ramgoolam A, Betz R, et al. Challenges to accessing pediatric health care in the Mississippi delta: a survey of emergency department patients seeking nonemergency care. J Prim Care Community Health 2010;1:152–7.

6. Berry E. Emergency department volumes rises as office visits fall. AMA News 2012.

7. Ragin DF, Hwang U, Cydulka RK, et al. Reasons for using the emergency department: results of the EMPATH Study. Acad Emerg Med 2005;12:1158–66.

8. Ginns P, Barrie S. Reliability of single-item ratings of quality in higher education: a replication. Psychol Rep 2004;95:1023–30.

9. Wanous JP, Hudy MJ. Single-item reliability: a replication and extension. Organ Res Meth 2001;4:361–75.

10. Powell-Young YM, Spruill IJ. Views of Black nurses toward genetic research and testing. J Nurs Scholarsh 2013;45:151–9.

11. Hines AL, Fraze T, Stocks C. Emergency Department Visits in Rural and Non-Rural Community Hospitals. HCUP Statistical Brief #116. June 2011. Rockville (MD): Agency for Healthcare Research and Quality; 2008. Available at: http://www.hcup-us.ahrq.gov/reports/statbriefs/sb116.pdf.

12. McWilliams A, Tapp H, Barker J, et al. Cost analysis of the use of emergency departments for primary care services in Charlotte, North Carolina. N C Med J 2011; 72:265–71.

13. Tang N, Stein J, Hsia RY, et al. Trends and characteristics of US emergency department visits, 1997-2007. JAMA 2010;304:664–70.

14. Gindi RM, Jones LI. Reasons for emergency room use among U.S. children: National Health Interview Survey, 2012. NCHS Data Brief 2014;(160):1–8.

15. Carret ML, Fassa AC, Domingues MR. Inappropriate use of emergency services: a systematic review of prevalence and associated factors. Cad Saude Publica 2009;25:7–28.

16. Griffey RT, Kennedy SK, McGownan L, et al. Is low health literacy associated with increased emergency department utilization and recidivism? Acad Emerg Med 2014;21:1109–15.

17. Schumacher JR, Hall AG, Davis TC, et al. Potentially preventable use of emergency services: the role of low health literacy. Med Care 2013;51:654–8.

18. van der Linden MC, Lindeboom R, van der Linden N, et al. Self-referring patients at the emergency department: appropriateness of ED use and motives for self-referral. Int J Emerg Med 2014;7:28. eCollection.

Index

Note: Page numbers of article titles are in **boldface** type.

Nurs Clin N Am 50 (2015) 621–629
http://dx.doi.org/10.1016/S0029-6465(15)00077-8
0029-6465/15/$ – see front matter © 2015 Elsevier Inc. All rights reserved.

nursing.theclinics.com

.

Printed and bound by CPI Group (UK) Ltd, Croydon, CR0 4YY

03/10/2024

01040497-0019